EATING
DANGEROUSLY

EATING
DANGEROUSLY

Why the Government Can't
Keep Your Food Safe . . .
and How You Can

Michael Booth and Jennifer Brown

ROWMAN & LITTLEFIELD

Lanham • Boulder • New York • Toronto • Plymouth, UK

Published by Rowman & Littlefield
4501 Forbes Boulevard, Suite 200, Lanham, Maryland 20706
www.rowman.com

10 Thornbury Road, Plymouth PL6 7PP, United Kingdom

Distributed by National Book Network

British Library Cataloguing in Publication Information Available

Library of Congress Cataloging-in-Publication Data

Booth, Michael, 1965–
  Eating dangerously : why the government can't keep your food safe—and how you can / Michael Booth and Jennifer Brown.
    pages cm
  Includes bibliographical references and index.
  ISBN 978-1-4422-2266-3 (cloth : alk. paper) — ISBN 978-1-4422-2267-0 (electronic)
  1. Food poisoning—United States—Prevention. 2. Food adulteration and inspection—Government policy—United States. 3. Food—Safety measures.
  I. Brown, Jennifer, 1975– II. Title.
  RA601.B66 2014
  615.9'45—dc23

                                                                    2013037125

∞™ The paper used in this publication meets the minimum requirements of American National Standard for Information Sciences—Permanence of Paper for Printed Library Materials, ANSI/NISO Z39.48-1992.

Printed in the United States of America

To our families, who are always the best reasons for cooking safely and eating well

CONTENTS

INTRODUCTION

For about six months while researching and writing this book, we became more than a little neurotic in the kitchen. We rinsed fruits even though we planned to peel them later. Hovered and commented while watching our families crack eggs into pancake mix. Stopped eating some troubled foods altogether. Grocery shopping induced mini bouts of panic: Is it better to buy the prewashed greens in bags, or the organic bunches that weren't stirred up with 10,000 pounds of other lettuces? Coworkers on lunch break learned to walk away when the conversation turned to poultry warehouses or what a norovirus outbreak looks like on a packed cruise ship.

As journalists at *The Denver Post*, we spent months covering the listeria outbreak linked to Colorado cantaloupe that killed thirty three people in 2011. The reporting turned into something of an obsession. Then we settled down and realized this was no way to eat, or to live. Wasn't there a way to cut down a few outsize risks without losing the joy of food and the satisfaction of sharing it with friends and family?

What we needed was what this book turned out to be: A clear explanation of some basic problems in our food safety system, followed by some succinct, practical advice on safety and the fast-changing near-future of food. We learned to stop worrying about every raw egg. Much easier just to wipe off the counter later with an antibacterial spray. We resumed eating shrimp.

But there were other pieces of advice gathered while researching this book that did stick. Our refrigerators, for example, are now set up to keep meat on the bottom, below the fresh produce that will be eaten raw. We no longer rinse raw chicken in the sink. And we each occasionally remember to toss reusable grocery bags in the washing machine. We hope that's what happens to you after you read this book—that you will absorb some things you didn't know and use what works for you. It's not intended to scare anyone away from food altogether. Think of it as steering you through the grocery aisles, not away from them.

Eating Dangerously isn't the final word on food safety. That's because it is difficult to put a period at the end of any sentence written about the subject. New outbreaks of foodborne illness happen weekly in America. In recent months alone, an outbreak of rare cyclospora linked to salads sickened hundreds in the Midwest— with infighting among state agencies over the speed of the investigation—and an *E. coli* outbreak from a Mexican restaurant in the Southwest put dozens at risk for kidney failure.

The FDA punctuates the bad news with optimistic new rules for safety improvements, then quickly acknowledges it hasn't nailed down the money to pay for progress. The point of this book is to provide an understanding of how the food safety net works, or doesn't, in America. In the second half of the book, we offer advice for keeping you and your family safer—what foods to avoid if you are particularly susceptible to foodborne illness, how to know when to call a doctor, and whether buying organic means you are any less likely to get sick. In the end, we hope we've proven to be good test cases for a rational consumer approach: skeptical, but not cynical; aware, but not hysterical.

I

SHOULD WE BE AFRAID OF OUR FOOD?

0

SICK: IT'S WHAT'S FOR DINNER

Americans are staring at their plates and wondering what lurks there.

Dying of a contaminated cantaloupe shouldn't rank high on a person's list of fears. Nor should bad spinach at a fast food restaurant, or undercooked hamburger, or eggs crawling with *Salmonella*. Yet every month seems to bring consumers a new food threat.

The cantaloupe your mom told you was the healthiest fruit, chock full of vitamins? It killed thirty-three people in 2011, the worst foodborne illness outbreak in one hundred years, on produce never before known to foster a bacteria called *Listeria*. Every deadly melon came from one Colorado family farm never before inspected by a government authority.[1] In 2012, another cantaloupe scare swept Eastern states, this time from *Salmonella*. In 2013, the Food and Drug Administration (FDA) warned cantaloupe farmers it was tired of the outbreaks and would send inspectors directly to their packing sheds.

That chicken fresh off the grill? It came in a package literally swimming in potentially lethal *Salmonella*, a fact known and approved by inspectors. Chicken factories find it too onerous to remove bacteria during their increasingly industrialized processing, so many plastic-wrapped packages of chicken come with *Salmonella*.[2] Federal regulators, squeezed by budget cuts and increasing production, are complicit in the gamble—they punt, and say it's up to the consumers to cook out the bacteria themselves.

A takeout taco from the Mexican place with the famous chihuahua? Even as dozens got sick around the nation from a *Salmonella* strain and state authorities found high numbers of those sickened had eaten at the ubiquitous taco shacks with the bell on the sign, federal and state officials refused to warn consumers by publicly broadcasting the name of the chain.[3]

Thinking of just sticking to the healthy stuff, like spinach? Producers are planning on irradiating it at the factory in the near future. That may be the good news. If they don't run it through the microwaves on the packaging line, you'll still have to worry about the safety of leafy greens in the American diet. Spinach, lettuce, and other "healthy" greens are known as some of the most stubborn carriers of food-illness pathogens, their porous surfaces vulnerable to a host of bacteria lurking in the soil of massive farms, in the runoff from nearby farms or ranches, and in the elaborate machinery of the sorting factories.

Horse meat in IKEA's famous meatballs. Hamburger patties in school cafeterias held together with a protein glue popularly dubbed "pink slime," infused by ammonia gas at the factory as a safety measure.[4] Today food moves around the globe with lightning speed. Traditional small producers consolidate into massive food-assembly operations. Geneticists alter the very DNA of what we're planning for dinner. Now more than ever, consumers need a reliable, rational gauge for judging food safety in a vast and confusing marketplace.

The problem is, consumers aren't getting those rational safety measures from their government. Nearly fifty million Americans will get food poisoning this year. That's one in six people who will get sick from something they ate. More than one hundred thousand will go to the hospital; three thousand will die.[5] The notorious cantaloupe *Listeria* outbreak in 2011 was the deadliest modern-day food poisoning event in America. But it was just one of dozens of multistate, foodborne illness outbreaks the Centers for Disease Control (CDC) and Prevention tracks in any given year. In 2013, two years after passage of a landmark food safety update by Congress meant to drag oversight into modern times, the CDC dimmed hopes with a grim update. Not only had progress against the major foodborne pathogens flattened in recent years, but cases of *Campylobacter* and the lesser-known *Vibrio* were rising sharply.[6]

As a swarm of federal and state agents swooped down on Colorado's previously unknown Jensen Farms in September 2011, seeking the culprit in what would grow to thirty-three deaths from one outbreak, the gaping holes in the nation's food safety net had their most dramatic exposure in a century. For example: How often do you think the average factory-volume farm is visited by an inspector with government authority, actually looking for food pathogens and how they might spread? Once a year? That's a bit optimistic. How about every three or four years? A reasonable expectation, but not close.

Try never.

Jensen Farms had never been swabbed by inspectors who had a license to stop illnesses, not in years of producing cantaloupes, onions, carrots, watermelons, and other produce shipped to dozens of states.[7]

Ironically, for consumers in the American Southwest, buying a cool cantaloupe during a hot, dusty summer is a way to feel connected to farming. Some families even plan their August trips around the peak of the melon harvest, Google-mapping their vacation routes to drive by their favorite roadside stand, or buying a case of ripe melon at the grocery store on their way to a mountain cabin.

What cantaloupe buyers did not know in 2011 was that the Jensen family was changing the way it worked with hopes of reaching a higher level in agribusiness. The Jensen brothers had planted enough orange melon to supply dozens of states with three hundred thousand cases. They'd bought a washing and sorting machine able to handle a high volume of produce during the compressed packing season and to answer a private auditor's worries about dirty fruit. The used machine had proven itself to be a workhorse with the farm produce it was designed for: potatoes. The Jensens switched the machine from raw potatoes, which are covered in dirt but always cooked at high heat before eating, to cantaloupes, rarely cleaned and eaten raw.[8] And, though none of the moves appear to have been made knowing cleanliness might be compromised, they set in motion a deadly series of mistakes, unmasking major holes in the food safety net.[9]

The classic melons marked with the aficionado's brand "Rocky Ford" were shipped to grocery stores across the country. The growers, the food inspectors, the national distributor, the grocery chains, the health-conscious consumer—none had a clue that a deadly strain of *Listeria* bacteria was along for the ride, lurking in the distinctive mottled crevasses of the cantaloupe rinds.

It was a piece of Jensen cantaloupe, prepared as comfort food for a retiree recovering from an illness, that sent Mike Hauser into a chest-heaving seizure and months of a near-vegetative coma. And it was the coma that devastated Hauser's big family, ruined a lifetime of meticulous finances, and pushed his grieving wife, Penny, to make a simple demand unlikely to ever get a response. "I just want him to wake up so I can apologize to him for serving him cantaloupe," Penny Hauser said, as Mike's once-hearty body was stretched and compressed by a ventilator every few seconds. Penny Hauser sat for weeks at her husband's bedside in a drab rehabilitation hospital in Denver, agonizing with her children over this infuriating question: How could a food touted as such a healthy part of the human diet arrive on her kitchen counter covered in deadly bacteria?[10] Mike Hauser died in early 2012.

Congress and the FDA want us to believe the chances of another Jensen Farms fiasco will diminish greatly when they begin in earnest the implementation of the 2011 Food Safety Modernization act. The first major overhaul of food oversight laws in decades, the act was lauded by lawmakers and some consumer groups for giving the FDA mandatory recall authority—many consumers were surprised to learn the FDA didn't already have authority to recall bad products. The act also gives extra oversight of imported food, and more power to write guidelines for farmers on the best ways to grow food.[11] The more optimistic regulators said that if the modernization act had been passed a few years earlier, the Jensen Farms outbreak might never have happened.

And yet, the corrosive power of partisan politics quickly proved a match for any momentum for decisive action brought on by highly publicized foodborne illnesses. Congressional budget cutters don't want to fund the extra money the new law's provisions will require. In fact, they don't even want to pay for the existing, stretched-thin system the act was supposed to replace. The sequestration mess hit the FDA in 2013, and officials predicted they would be forced to give up 2,100 food inspection visits—talk of an actual budget increase fell to a distant whisper.[12] An act of Congress suggesting the FDA should now inspect all farms is powerless if there is no money to write tougher growing guidelines or to hire actual inspectors.

In the government's first budget cycle after the Jensen outbreak, the Obama administration's proposed budget increase for the FDA relied on new fees for food growers that Congress had already rejected in previous years.[13] Buried in other budget documents was news the administration had also proposed eliminating the only federal program to conduct swab bacterial tests on produce before it is shipped to consumers. It was a tiny, $5 million program, yet it had successfully weeded out contaminated food.[14]

Some consumer advocates are disturbed by other trends that appear to showcase the power of food companies and a growing deferential streak in their government watchdogs.

You may not know which Mexican food stand the government is talking about when it issues a warning about "Restaurant Chain A," but chances are you've been there on a late-night salsa run or hosted a postgame soccer team meal on the plastic-mold tabletops. In the fall of 2011, dozens of reports of *Salmonella enteritidis* in ten states eventually bubbled up to the level of the CDC and FDA. Pinpointing one type of food proved tricky in this case, because victims answering state health departments' traditional, long-form eating questionnaire reported a wide range of meals, restaurants, and ingredients.

As more and more victims with matching strains of *Salmonella* emerged from New Mexico to Michigan, the CDC set its vast computer database to work. The computer knows the eating habits of thousands of Americans who have filled out extensive questionnaires on what they eat, where they eat it, and who prepares it. The CDC quickly gathered that more than 60 percent of the ill people in this outbreak had recently eaten at "Chain A," while only 17 percent of healthy people eat at that chain in the average week. That's the kind of statistical anomaly epidemiologists notice. Researchers couldn't pin it down further, because Chain A—and all other fast food Mexican cafes—mix and match lettuce, cheese, meat, salsas, and tortillas in seemingly endless combinations. In this case, the ground beef got a rare pass from suspicions, since the CDC knew "Chain A" had an updated and approved meat-handling system. Eventually, investigators concluded the *Salmonella* must have come from a lower-level supplier of a handful of possible culprit foods, shipping to many states—but there was no question that most of the cases emanated from this famous chain.[15]

And that's all the public would know. The CDC refused to share the name of the chain, saying the tainted food was gone and there was no need to taint the name of the chain in turn. Yet it was the fourth significant outbreak from that chain in a few years, following *E. coli* in contaminated lettuce and two *Salmonella* outbreaks in 2010 that made 155 people sick in twenty-one states. Only the Oklahoma authorities, months later, were willing to reveal to the public what many already suspected, that "Chain A" was Taco Bell. Even after Oklahoma opened its books, the federal CDC stayed mum.[16] Taco Bell's response to journalists' questions was that the CDC had never narrowed the suspect food down to one item, and that not all victims had eaten at the company's restaurants.

Wouldn't fast food fans like to know what chains have a bad habit of hosting foodborne illnesses? Wouldn't local restaurant inspectors like to know which kitchens might deserve special attention? Wouldn't investors demand to hear what publicity challenges a multinational parent company faces? Wouldn't company executives endeavor to improve their supply chain under intense public scrutiny? The government increasingly decides no, consumer advocates say. Seattle food safety litigator Bill Marler calls it a "general withdrawal from the obligations of open disclosure," and many of his attempts to fight the silence have been ignored.[17]

Where does that leave the consumer who is striving to stay safe when it comes to family meals, yet who doesn't have the time or energy to study food safety, which would amount to a full-time job?

An overview of other notorious illness outbreaks in recent years offers more lessons in what big business and the government are not doing, and where we as shoppers and cooks might need to pick up the slack.

The clean, chilled rack of egg cartons at your local grocery store doesn't tell much of the story of modern chicken farming. Erase the image of a bucolic family garden with a few plump brown hens scratching around the yard. Now replace it with twelve to fifteen million chickens stacked beak to claw in warehouses bursting at the seams with overflowing manure, and you'll have a more realistic picture of where most Americans get their eggs. Industrial-strength chicken production leads to a by-product of multinational illness outbreaks. In 2010, somewhere in the middle of nearly two thousand people getting *Salmonella* across the nation, investigators descended on a massive chicken operation called Wright County Egg and a sister operation, Hillandale Farms, in Iowa. They found horror-show material.[18] Decaying mice, chicken carcasses, and flies "too numerous to count." Manure piled so high, the chicken-house door wouldn't shut.[19] More manure spilling into creeks running through the farm property. The volume of putrid waste created by such enormous farms was a vivid reminder to consumers of where much of their food is produced. As Wright and Hillandale began their recalls, the scale seemed even more overwhelming: eventually more than a half-billion eggs shipped from the company's farms would be called back, from just one outbreak investigation. As the company's reputation slowly unraveled through investigations, congressional hearings, and reports in the media that dripped with outrage, it also became clear the farms were repeat offenders of industry standards and food safety rules. Congressional investigators learned the farms had more than four hundred positive tests for *Salmonella* between 2008 and 2010.[20] Yet somehow the federal government either didn't know that, or didn't care enough to order changes. Egg and poultry operations have grown so massive in the United States, it stretches the imagination to comprehend how much danger emanates from just one company. When their 2010 troubles were finally winding down, Hillandale and Wright County Egg had together recalled 550 million eggs.

Even when we learn growers and producers aren't shipping us clean food, we usually assume the grocery store chains are looking out for us. It's their name on the shopping bag, after all. It's their reputation most at risk with consumers who will quickly turn elsewhere to put food on their table. So what about the grocers who bought millions of the tainted eggs every day from one of the leading producers in the United States? Didn't they want to know if the eggs were clean enough to sell? They claim they tried, with grocers and distributors hiring so-called third-party auditors to inspect the farms and certify their handling practices. Just how ineffective those audits turned out to be is now an ironic stain in the public record: Wright County boasted an embossed audit report labeled "superior," issued just before the company's eggs started sickening a couple of thousand people in a dozen states.[21]

Maybe it's with such messy conditions in mind that government officials and consumer experts throw up their hands at poultry products, telling consumers to assume there's *Salmonella* involved every time they handle them. Many home cooks know they are not supposed to eat raw eggs, either in a Caesar dressing or in cake batter. At the same time, federal officials give an official pass to poultry packers—people should expect that raw chicken parts in shrink-wrapped grocery packages are floating in a bath of *Salmonella*.

Many consumers shop for chicken and egg products without a clue their government and the poultry conglomerates are so blasé about shipping *Salmonella*. Shoppers believe someone else is policing the kitchen—often to their own peril.

And it's not just chicken and eggs we have to worry about.

Madison Sedbrook was only a kindergartener in 2009 when she nearly died after snacking on raw cookie dough. She was celebrating her big sister's return home from college, sampling a popular dough straight from the kind of tub many consumers keep in the back of the fridge for just such occasions.

Within days of eating the dough, the Colorado kid was "white as a sheet," lethargic and vomiting every thirty minutes. Madison was on the verge of kidney failure when doctors determined *E. coli* bacteria was the cause of her bloody diarrhea and violent nausea. Her mom, Cindy, recalls the chill of the doctors' description: Madison's blood had begun to clump, making it nearly impossible for her kidneys to function.[22]

CDC investigators called Cindy every two days to question her about her daughter's diet. Mostly, they asked about fruits and vegetables, because those are more common places where *E. coli* lurks, but they never inquired about cookie dough. Cindy even purchased another package of the dough after Madison had gotten ill—what could be more comforting to a child just home from the hospital than a home-baked cookie?

Madison battled the infection caused by *E. coli* for about a month, recovering just in time to attend kindergarten graduation and a ballet recital. The official CDC investigation never pinpointed just one ingredient in the raw cookie dough, although a later scientific study concluded that flour, of all things, was the most likely culprit.[23]

That outbreak of 2009 was the first time the CDC had linked the deadly *E. coli* O157:H7—the same strain implicated in the notorious Jack in the Box tainted beef of the early 1990s—to raw cookie dough. For many Americans, if they weren't already turned off by warnings about *Salmonella* in raw eggs, the episode ended the consumption of factory-made cookie dough straight out of the package. More than seventy people nationwide fell ill.[24] As with many highly publicized outbreaks, the bad cookie dough pushed consumers to look more skeptically at many things they used to eat with impunity. The Sedbrooks learned their lesson just a little too late. Somewhere in Madison's tenuous recovery from near organ failure, her dad looked in the fridge at his house, where Madison lived part time, and found another bucket of the once-tempting dough.

What's worrisome about the tainted cookie dough and the bad eggs and the dangerous cantaloupes, in addition to the illnesses they caused, is that, in a way, they represent success stories. Regulators found the problems in those particular foods and began doing something about them. But the government shows a troubling lack of resolve and resources when they have the chance to truly clean up after a major outbreak. Very few of the people and companies pinpointed in outbreak investigations ever suffer much more than bad publicity, no matter how rank the details in the inspection reports.

Consumers in nearly every state got sick in 2008 and 2009 from nuts traced to Peanut Corporation of America (PCA). Nine people died. Much of the company's enormous volume of nuts went into peanut butter sold in large tubs to schools and cafeterias. PCA nuts eventually recalled were in some four thousand different products, from granola bars to ice cream.[25] Health food enthusiasts paid a price as well. Thinking they were sidestepping harmful processors by turning raw peanuts into peanut butter with the turn of a handle at high-end grocery stores, they were actually crushing PCA nuts tainted with *Salmonella*.[26]

Investigators found PCA had a shocking disregard for the consumers at the other end of their production line. Congressional staffers unveiled emails in public hearings showing that company executives discussed internal lab results showing heaps of the peanuts were tainted and potentially poisonous.[27] When a plant manager said tainted product had been shipped and customers should hold off using the peanuts until they could get results from retests, the company president wrote back, "The time lapse . . . is costing us huge $$$$$." The company sought more favorable retests on the product from other labs, ignoring the proconsumer adage of "when in doubt, throw it out." Other emails hammered home what U.S. Representative Bart Stupak of Michigan called "a total systemic breakdown" in the company and the regulators whose job it was to oversee safety.[28] When retests came back negative on the same peanuts, the same company chief wrote, "Turn them loose."[29]

PCA was also tested by third-party auditors to assure buyers the company's leaky, rodent-infested warehouses were actually safe. The results of those audits, just before the *Salmonella* outbreak? Another batch of certificates featuring the word *superior*.

Victims of the families hurt by the bad peanut butter say the PCA case points out another glaring flaw in the U.S. food safety system: lack of consequences for any of the companies at ground zero of the outbreaks. Jeff Almer's mother, in Minnesota, was one of the nine known to have died from the peanut butter *Salmonella*. Almer sat at congressional hearings on PCA and felt his sorrow over his mother transform into raw fury when staffers revealed the internal company emails, appearing to have pushed tainted product out the door to consumers. He said later he wondered why company president Stewart Parnell faced no criminal consequences more than three years after the outbreak, despite a long FBI and FDA probe. "I don't know how much clearer you can be. It's hard to fathom what's taking so damn long," Almer said.[30]

PCA went bankrupt. Parnell and other company employees were finally charged with federal crimes in 2013, and as of now are awaiting a trial. In the meantime, news reports noted Parnell had since found other work. As a consultant. To the peanut industry.[31]

The dangers to our health when farmers and regulators get it wrong are obvious. But each outbreak also threatens the reputation of an entire category of food, and all the jobs and commerce that go with it. Consumer reaction to food safety news has been revolutionized by the penetration of twenty-four-hour news outlets, and the unstoppable social power of the Internet. Rarely has that manifested in a shelf-clearing food panic as rapid as in the leafy greens scare of 2006.

Within a week's time in September 2006, consumers across the country started hearing vague reports of people falling dreadfully ill with a strain of *E. coli*; then reports that many of the victims had eaten bagged fresh spinach; then, suddenly, a stark warning from the FDA that the public "should not eat fresh spinach or fresh spinach-containing products." After decades of being told to eat those mighty greens for health, Americans were now being told nutritious spinach was toxic. Victims were going into kidney failure, which of course means a lifetime of tedious and uncomfortable dialysis, along with other health threats. The impact on U.S. eating habits was stark: salad bars had gaping holes, and whole sections of grocery store produce departments had bare shelves. The storied name of Dole didn't seem quite so fresh. By winter, a separate *E. coli* outbreak traced largely to restaurants was eventually linked to greens from the same part of agriculture-rich central California that had produced the spinach. The Central Valley, one of the wealthiest and most powerful agricultural engines in the nation, was reeling.[32]

Yet the response of the California agricultural powers has been one of the rare bright spots in food safety in recent years, and it could shine the light for other food producers struggling to prove to consumers their products are still safe. California state officials worked with federal outbreak investigators to drill deep into the leafy green illness cases and Central Valley farms' extensive records. They soon isolated the bad spinach to one fifty-acre farm, and the likeliest *E. coli* source as the next-door Angus cattle ranch. Irrigation water apparently washed across the cattle manure, commonly tainted with the bacteria dangerous to humans, and onto the greens.[33]

Grocery stores terrified of losing their salad business ordered farmers to come up with a new safety plan. Farmers banded together with state agriculture officials to create their own mandatory inspection plan, funded by farm fees and grounded in random bacterial swab testing. Shipments were held until specific tests on those lots came back negative, a gold standard for food safety that produce providers had previously resisted as unworkable.

With consumers shunning salad and farmers losing hundreds of millions of dollars off their traditional sales levels—from just one item in the salad bar—there was little choice but to create a whole new layer of food safety for California. The scale of food production in the state has simply grown too large for an antiquated regulatory system. According to news reports at the time, the Golden State had 120,000 farms and food-processing plants in 2006. Overseeing them all were three inspectors from the state and thirty from the FDA.[34] Now the state produce system appears to be much safer to most outside experts, and in the wake of the *Listeria* outbreak, it was California cantaloupe growers who took the lead in restoring consumer confidence with new safety measures. They'd watched their farm brethren strive to revive the California greens brand after 2006, and they had taken careful notes.

It's hard to call the exact year when Americans started to take a closer look at their dinner plates and began to consider more seriously whether the food there was safe. With so many seminal outbreak events, it's a challenge to choose the one that most changed the U.S. consumer food mindset. But a prime candidate is the Jack in the Box *E. coli* food poisonings of 1993, which put a target on all fast food and launched an overhaul of the meat industry that was long the most stubborn force resisting any kind of food safety change.[35]

When diners started getting sick in Northwestern states that year, epidemiologists quickly rolled through their protocols of isolating the suspect food. They learned many of the victims had eaten hamburger patties, and repeat interviews and cross-checking found many of those had been at the regional Jack in the Box chain. Four children died. At key points in the outbreak, investigators found their hands tied: the particularly virulent strain of *E. coli* they were dealing with, O157:H7, wasn't considered an official "adulterant." That meant there were no rules against shipping raw hamburger containing the bacteria. The consumer-unfriendly rule at the time was "cook it to clean it." In other words, it was the cook's job to battle the bacteria with heat and make sure internal temperatures reached high enough to destroy the pathogen before someone ate the burger.

Jack in the Box resisted blame for a while and pointed fingers in many other directions. The supplier. Other restaurants. But the chain also announced a revamping of all its cooking procedures to ensure hamburger patties reached the ideal bacteria-killing temperatures. It all seemed like a big mistake, quickly rectified by a homegrown restaurant chain.

But a Seattle law firm representing many of the sickened victims didn't like to take the word of company executives at face value. The lawyers asked for proof, in the form of long depositions and daunting hours of document discovery. They had the power to keep asking, through the rules of liability lawsuits and the leverage of money from previous big judgments that paid for costly research. Attorney Bill Marler's team found the *E. coli* burgers were not just a mistake from a broken grill thermometer or an inattentive fry cook. They uncovered internal memos showing Jack in the Box employees were intentionally shorting the cooking time because the company thought temperatures recommended by local health departments left their burgers too tough.[36]

The outrage was swift, expensive, and transformative in the beef industry. Marler obtained a $15 million settlement for just one of his clients. The FDA raised its cooked-beef recommendations for restaurants to 155 degrees. (The home-cooked consumer standard is actually higher, at a 160-degree internal target.) And federal officials finally added the most danger-

ous strains of *E. coli* to the official "adulterants" list, meaning meat processors and other middlemen could be liable just for shipping beef tainted by
the bacteria. It was no longer the sole burden of consumers to cook their
burgers to safety. The meat has to be clean when it leaves the factory floor.[37]

But the food factories are a stubborn lot.

Remember all that *Salmonella* floating around inside the packages of
processed poultry? It's still legal. It's not the chicken factory's job to ship
you a clean bird. You're supposed to assume the pathogen is there, at $4.99
a pound, and cook it out for yourself. Shouldn't the worst strains of *Salmonella* be official "adulterants" too? Almost twenty years after Jack in the Box
was a national pariah, the government is still debating that one.

2

TOO MANY COOKS,
NOT ENOUGH TEST TUBES

When stomachs start heaving, fingers start pointing.

A foodborne illness outbreak hits the news, and a familiar blame game begins. State health officials pinpoint the farm or the factory or the distributor where the food safety chain was broken. That's where it all began, they announce to media hungry for answers. The farm blames the auditor it hired to ensure safe handling, arguing, "They never told us to fix that—we got perfect scores!" The auditor says it's just taking a snapshot of how things looked for one hour of one day, and they never meant to guarantee long-term safety. The questions turn toward the grocery store—shouldn't the large chain with the deep pockets pay for a strict food safety audit with mandatory follow-up checks? The grocery store responds that the consumer demands cheap food and won't pay the higher prices it would take to finance top-notch audits. Watchdog groups want to know why audits and government inspections don't include more microbe testing of actual product, and why products aren't sequestered on hold until the tests come back negative. And everybody blames the government for failing to send out enough of its own independent inspectors, and for missing rulemaking deadlines by years at a time when new guidelines could have prevented new outbreaks.[1]

So who is responsible? Who guarantees safe food for U.S. kitchens and pantries? Are we wrong for assuming adults are in charge?

The answers are as multilayered as peeling the husk away from sweet corn. Let's say you bought a melon at a roadside stand. Chances are that farm has never been inspected by government authorities.[2] If you bought the whole melon at a chain grocery store, there's a good chance the farm had to hire a "third-party auditor" to assure the chain store that the farm used good practices. But that doesn't mean the auditor ever sampled the farm's operations for bacteria, or even required the producer to make corrections of obvious hazards. If you bought the melon as cut-up fruit salad inside a plastic package, the FDA may have visited that production plant to check on the process. But budget cutters and industry opponents keep attacking the few government-run testing programs that would have swabbed those melon packs for pathogens.[3]

But who is in charge of which foods?

If you bought beef in a package, then a U.S. Department of Agriculture inspector reported to work in that plant every single day.

But eggs bought in the grocery store are the FDA's responsibility.

Then again, liquid-egg safety is back at the USDA.

Chicken meat is the USDA's problem.

But ostrich and emu meat? FDA.[4]

Rabbit meat? FDA. Duck meat? USDA.

Catfish? USDA. Flounder? FDA.

Those of you seeking safe goat meat, flip a coin, it's got to be one of those agencies or the other.

This bewildering crosshatch of occasional oversight can leave the consumer with an impression from a distance that all these agencies add up to a tight safety net. Federal food safety duties are split among fifteen different agencies, according to the Congressional Research Service. But moving closer to see how food actually moves through the system makes the holes look wider and wider. It doesn't help that food production has grown as mysterious to us as the microchips inside our cell phones, or the wiring that keeps an airliner aloft. Each time an outbreak is traced back to one farm or one handling plant, naïve Americans must remind ourselves exactly how far most of us are removed from our agricultural roots. When we ask why someone wasn't standing over a farmer's shoulders, testing every batch before it got shipped, we reveal our growing ignorance of the food system at a time when fewer than 1 percent of us claim farming as an occupation. As many farmers and food marketers remind us continually throughout our research, food is still grown in dirt. Dirt is still enriched by fertilizer, whether animal manure or petroleum based. Birds, deer, mice, and countless insects still cross open fields, doing all kinds of business along the way. Let's try not to create the impression as city slickers that we expect every morsel of food to endure a chlorine bath before gracing our plates.

There were 2,800 food-related employees at the FDA in 2011, responsible for the oversight of 350,000 food makers, food facilities, and food importers.[5] Grocery stores and farms make up the oversight gap, in nearly every fresh item besides meat and eggs, by hiring third-party auditors to assess the safety of their methods. The arrangements often leave just enough room for that fingerpointing to break out with every breakout. Costco, for example, doesn't necessarily hire the auditors directly. The warehouse chain offers suppliers a list of about nine approved auditors whose reports it will accept out of hundreds of such auditing outfits around the nation.[6] The actual hiring of the auditor is done by the farm, producer or a distributor—grocery chains have long tried to avoid issuing ironclad food safety guarantees under the stamp of their own audits. They instead want the farm and the auditor and the distributor who brought them the produce to take responsibility for what they've just delivered.

The farm has no choice but to get an auditor with most grocery store or distributor contracts. They are a given. But the farm is also operating on razor-thin margins and is constantly under the threat of a preharvest rain, a sudden shortage in pickers, or dozens of other daily miseries on a farmer's worry list. Farm operators often don't have the time or the money to choose an auditor who has experience in cantaloupes, say, or a deep background in raw potatoes. Auditors offer varying levels of review[7]—which level do you think the farmer will most likely sign for, after being squeezed by Costco, Walmart, Kroger, and other chains to cram down prices as far as possible?

Jensen Farms signed up for what amounted to a checklist audit in 2011 when it was trying out new systems to speed cantaloupe production for its contract with Southwestern distributor Frontera Produce. The auditor, BioFood Safety, had a friendly relationship with Jensen, and in 2010 it had even offered advice on how to expand the Southeastern Colorado farm. In 2011, BioFood Safety sent a young man two years out of college, with two one-week training courses on food audits. Executives couldn't say whether he'd ever had any experience on a cantaloupe farm.[8]

There on page 1 of the audit is the phrase the FDA, congressional investigators, and food safety experts say was key to the deaths of at least thirty-three people from cantaloupe in the Jensen Farms outbreak: "No antimicrobial solution is injected into the water of the wash station."[9] In other words, Jensen cantaloupes were not dumped into a chlorine-enhanced bath before workers packed them in shipping boxes. That was the fateful switch for 2011, in the eyes of all critics. The Jensens later told Congress they believed their new system for 2011 was even safer: a one-pass cleaning shower using continual fresh water, instead of cantaloupes swimming in a bath of chlorine and dirt with the sanitizer under constant threat of being overwhelmed by field bacteria.

The FDA's inspection and report to the public in the fall of 2011 were brutal on the Jensens.[10] Water that tested positive for *Listeria* was pooling on the farm's conveyor belts, on the floor around sorting areas, and in trenches meant to drain dirty liquids. The main cantaloupe sorter was actually a potato machine, designed for a food usually blasted by four hundred degrees of heat for up to an hour before being eaten. These cantaloupes, of course, were to be eaten raw, and FDA investigators found dirt and water building up throughout the mismatched potato machinery. After sorting on the dangerous machinery, the Jensens took another chance by placing boxes straight into cold storage. Cantaloupe farms are supposed to "precool" the big fruit, so their still-hot, wet rinds don't sit steaming in storage while bacteria multiply, according to FDA standards and industry practice. By the time congressional staff interviewed the FDA a few weeks later, the government was laying the deaths even closer to the feet of the Jensens: agency officials told the Energy and Commerce Committee "the outbreak could have likely been prevented if Jensen Farms had maintained its facilities in accordance with existing FDA guidance."[11]

Wonderful fodder for lawsuits. But not quite fair in the grand scheme of fingerpointing. Though the FDA made it sound otherwise, its existing "guidance" on growing cantaloupes did not require or even strongly suggest a bleaching agent in the fruit wash. In fact, the 2009 guidance in effect that fateful summer warned of dirt overwhelming the sanitizer in large melon baths, and it suggested a single pass through clean water might do the trick.[12]

And one would assume given the urgency of thirty-three deaths and the weight of the worst foodborne illness outbreak in a century that the FDA would rush to update all its produce guidance. The Food Safety and Modernization Act signed into law in early 2011 legislatively guaranteed such a rush, setting mandated deadlines for all sorts of new rules. And yet by late fall of 2012, the new rules were stuck in bureaucratic purgatory. They sat in the Office of Management and Budget, with food safety groups suing the government to pry them loose. One watchdog called it an unlawful "abdication" that with every day of delay was "putting millions of lives at risk."[13]

The third-party audit commissioned by the Jensens did note a few "major deficiencies," despite the excellent final score of 96 percent. There was no hot water at the hand-washing stations for employees sorting and packing the cantaloupes, for example. And packing shed doors to the outside were left wide open, leaving room for pests to join the packing party. Surely the auditor returned later to make sure the deficiencies were corrected?[14]

That's not the way the auditing system works, though, in the great majority of smaller food operations. Follow-up costs extra. A lot extra. A "checklist" audit fills the paperwork requirement of the distributors and buyers and may never be seen by anyone but the farm and the auditor filing it. A higher-intensity audit where deficiencies are posted online for buyers to see, and which are not checked off until corrected and verified by a return visit, can cost thousands of dollars more.[15] Besides, is the auditor ever going to be tough enough on the farm when the farm is the one paying the auditing bill? It's the fox guarding the hen house, and the packing shed, and the water supply, and the cold storage. "There is a long and storied history of food safety failures involving third-party audits," according to a 2012 report in the journal *Food Control* led by Kansas State University researcher Douglas Powell.[16] Democrats issuing a minority report for the congressional committee investigating the Jensen Farms outbreak concluded, "There are inherent conflicts of interest with the third-party auditor relationship . . . we believe reforms in third-party audits are essential."

And none of this criticism of "checklist" audits gets to the question of testing actual products for dangerous microbes. A paper audit will tell you if a farm has a plan, and if it followed the plan. It will not say if the farm's product is safe to eat. It's like telling airline passengers as they strap into their seats: "This is your Captain speaking. The airplane you're sitting in was designed by professionals. We're pretty sure the people who built it used the blueprints. But it hasn't actually been in the air yet. That would have cost extra."

No one is arguing that every individual cantaloupe, every leaf of spinach, every package of sprouts should get its own dab on a petri dish to check for pathogens before sale. There aren't enough dollars, enough technicians, enough labs to perform such pathogen tests item for item, and time delays would spoil most produce before it ever got to market. But there are companies who are using past failures to craft strict testing regimens that help them prove whether their safety plans are written and executed effectively.

"Test and hold" is one of the most sacred food safety mantras at California's Earthbound Farm, a big organic player in the valley that supplies the majority of greens to U.S. consumers. Earthbound Farm believes so strongly in test and hold, it does it twice. Raw greens coming in from the field, whether grown on owned fields or by a partner supplier, are sampled for pathogens and sequestered until lab tests come back negative, according to company officials. Once spinach and other greens are sorted, washed, and packaged for shipping to the public, batches are once again sample tested and held until labs come back negative. Despite ongoing produce industry protests that those test-and-hold strategies aren't realistic given the short shelf life of fruits and vegetables, Earthbound Farm swears by it, and its strength in the marketplace only seems to grow.[17]

Such transparency is a matter of survival for Earthbound and other central California growers, who were nearly wiped out by the 2006 *E. coli* scare that emptied grocery store shelves of bagged spinach. Long before that scandal threatened the greens industry, Earthbound executives thought they were already out front of their peers in food safety. One vice president had noticed in the late 1990s a disturbing pattern in the company's third-party audits: the workers always knew when the auditors were coming, and they cleaned up accordingly. For a time. Then, a few weeks after the announced audit had passed, Earthbound operations slipped back to a more casual, everyday state. So food safety chief Will Daniels made all audits into surprise visits. The results were common sense: when workers from the bagging lines up to the executive offices had no idea when the auditors would show up, suddenly every day was Food Safety Day. And that's the way it should be for consumer goods, Daniels argues.

That wasn't enough to save bagged spinach in 2006. Reports started trickling into doctors' offices and state health departments of patients scattered throughout the nation, suffering the bloody diarrhea, severe cramps and intestinal distress, and nascent kidney failure of the worst strains of *E. coli* infection. From a public health "cluster" in Wisconsin, statistics mounted until two hundred people were sickened by a matching strain of *E. coli*, and 30 percent of those had severe kidney malfunction. Three died.

Food consumption questionnaires reduced the likely transmission to salad greens. Investigators found leftover bags of spinach in patients' refrigerators, tested for matching *E. coli*, and then traced most of the bags back to one supplier in central California—Earthbound. The company put out its own products such as "Natural Selection," while it also bagged produce under contract for household names such as Dole.[18] Federal and California scientists descended on the farm, swabbing and analyzing conveyors, washers, baggers, and shipping areas. Failing to find *E. coli* after days of customary sanitizing of the equipment, they went farther afield. Literally. Spinach cutting and hauling machines tested negative. So the probe went to the ground. Labs took field samples of creek water, stray animal feces, and just plain dirt from ranches surrounding Earthbound where cattle fattened near spinach rows. The results are catalogued in state reports using overhead photographs and pinpoint charting, as if a U2 spy plane were seeking hidden nuclear silos: the deadly *E. coli* strain had started on the ranch. They could never say exactly how it got into the spinach, but the possibilities were many. The final report features pictures of cattle wading through muddy streams near the spinach, and well-preserved hoof prints of wild pigs that likely dragged pathogens all over the ranch fields.

Ashlee Litkey has read those reports, and she remains deeply frustrated that they don't offer a full explanation of the tainted spinach that sickened her to the point that doctors told her parents to prepare themselves for her death. Litkey was a budding nursing school student with a new boyfriend the week before Labor Day 2006. She was to start nursing classes in Milwaukee the next week, and she had just moved into a school dorm. On Thursday, she had diarrhea and nausea, and she thought it was the meat from the tacos she'd made with her boyfriend, Cody. By Saturday, she couldn't eat. By Sunday, her diarrhea turned bloody, and while a thorough health education had left her finely tuned to the dangerous progression of symptoms, she was between work and student insurance and reluctant to even go to an ER. Relatives and friends eventually talked her into going to a hospital, where nurses took a stool sample and gave her an IV drip, but sent her home. On Monday, she couldn't walk. An ER doctor made her check into the hospital. On Tuesday, the stool sample came back positive for *E. coli*, though she wouldn't learn of the source for weeks. She was soon in renal failure, with terrifying symptoms of ICU psychosis. An EEG showed slowing of her brain function, and doctors said she had no better than a 50 percent chance of survival. In mid-September, state health officials told her family other patients' lab tests had narrowed the culprit food to spinach. Always a health-conscious eater, Litkey was shocked. "I ate spinach every single day, and I'd never heard of greens doing that," she said.[19]

Two weeks in the ICU and a month in the hospital, Litkey finally began to recover, but her weight swung through fluid gains and losses from 98 pounds to 148 pounds and back to 93. At Halloween, she was well enough to see friends, but she was not energetic enough to party. "I fell asleep on the couch at 9 p.m., in my Audrey Hepburn costume," she said. She didn't begin her nursing classes until February. "I tried eating spinach soon after that, in an artichoke dip, and had a panic attack after one bite," she said.

As she and her kidneys slowly recovered, Litkey finished nursing school and married Cody. More than $350,000 in hospital bills were paid by a legal settlement negotiated by the Seattle firm Marler Clark, and the couple received additional money as protection against an uncertain future. "We don't have a lot of long-term *E. coli* studies," said Litkey, who now lives

in Austin. "They can't say what will happen to me when I'm sixty-five"—
whether she'll be able to work, whether her once-weakened kidneys will
need dialysis. She ignored initial doctor's advice about avoiding the strain
of having children, and she gave birth to a healthy baby in 2012. She won't
eat bagged salads, and she avoids produce from central California, knowing
it's more superstition than fact. "There's only so much I can do to be safe,"
she said. She's incredulous that the Obama administration let the only federal produce testing program die, and she constantly battles the food safety
ignorance of well-meaning friends or relatives who think, say, that raw milk
is more wholesome than a factory-treated product.

Reminders of her near-death, tainted-food experience are hard to
avoid. Just after her lawsuit was settled, Litkey got a letter from Sam's
Club. Seems that she had bought granola bars containing peanut butter
from the 2009 peanut *Salmonella* scandal. Too late. "I'd eaten them all
already," she said.[20]

Two weeks after the spinach outbreak was traced to its doorstep, Earthbound Farm revolutionized its food safety program. The company had long
floated leafy greens in a wash permeated with a sanitizer that killed more
than 99 percent of bacteria, but as in all leafy green plants, a full "kill step"
would have required so much bleaching the greens would have been ined-
ible. So "test and hold" took over: test a sample of incoming raw greens,
and hold them as raw until tests cleared the batch. Then sort, wash, and
package. And test and hold again: the shipment doesn't leave until samples
from the packaged batch come back negative for pathogens.[21]

The new strategy doesn't guarantee every single leaf in every single bag is
bacteria free, Earthbound notes. No workable testing regimen can do that.
The produce industry and many reputable university scientists dismiss the
concept of apple-by-apple or stalk-by-stalk testing as an unattainable, neurotic ideal. "The FDA has said on multiple occasions you can't test your way
to safe food," said David Gombas, a microbiologist and food safety expert
with United Fresh Produce, an industry group based in Washington, D.C.[22]

Even microbe-testing believers like Earthbound know the limitations of
their faith in labs. "But it's another hurdle in a multi-hurdle approach we
take," Daniels said. "It's designed to catch gross contamination events. We
built it around our example. If the government investigation of us was correct, we processed five hundred pounds from the implicated field on that
day, a very small amount. And we processed tens of thousands of pounds
overall on that day; so only five hundred pounds led to that outbreak." Or
as another produce industry biologist put it, "That was five acres of spinach

that shut down the entire industry for a month." Six months after people stopped getting ill, spinach sales were still down as much as 50 percent.

Throughout the 2006 spinach scare, and the 2009 peanut debacle, and the 2010 egg scandal, and the 2011 *Listeria* tragedy, there was one government program that did send inspectors out to swab food for sale in real time and to get results in a petri dish while the product was still on the shelf.

The Microbiological Data Program (MDP) is a little-known federal testing regimen that serves as the "mall cop" of U.S. food security—ignored by most, disrespected even by the few who know about it, and yet protecting real consumers from real harm. A tiny office in the U.S. Department of Agriculture, the MDP paid state labs to pull samples of the most troublesome produce in the American palate: bagged lettuce and spinach, sprouts, cantaloupes, small tomatoes, cilantro, and more. The program grows cultures overnight and occasionally identified deadly pathogens like *Listeria*, *Salmonella*, and *E. coli* strains, contributing to numerous recalls. But it also detailed patterns of problems that could help growers, packers, and distributors with big-picture changes improving all of their food safety systems. And it brought technology and incomparable experience to the eleven states most heavily involved, honing their skills to more quickly zero in on other unrelated outbreaks, such as the Jensen Farms cantaloupe investigation.[23]

In fact, the summer after the deadly Jensen Farms outbreak, a routine product test carried out by the MDP led to the recall of an entire growing season from Burch Farms of North Carolina, shipments that reached from Maine to Florida and west to Ohio. The bacteria found by the random samplings? *Listeria*. The fruit involved? Cantaloupe and honeydew.[24]

The USDA's program conducted thirty-five thousand biological tests in 2011 alone, representing 80 percent of all government produce sampling at any level. It was a little program with a big punch, working to keep the food industry honest on a budget of a few million dollars a year. The cantaloupe deaths had raised food safety concerns to a new level in Washington, coming on the heels of revelatory congressional hearings on bad eggs and bad peanuts. President Obama himself had made the connection between farm and fork, remarking that his kids went through periods of virtually living on peanut butter and that neither he nor any American parent should have to worry about them getting sick from such a common food. He publicly vowed a complete review of FDA standards and practices.[25]

And yet while reports of deaths from the Jensen Farms cantaloupes were still trickling in, Obama's next budget proposal dropped the MDP altogether. The annual cost of the doomed testing program? Less than

$5 million a year. Elsewhere in the president's same budget, the FDA unknowingly underlined just how bad a bargain it will turn out to be for Americans: preventing just one death from *E. coli* saves $7 million.[26]

Much as they wanted to preserve the only nationwide testing program for farm goods, food safety advocates were even more concerned that the most important overhaul of U.S. food rules since the 1930s would never really get off the ground. The Food Safety Modernization Act of 2011 promised progress in a few long-sought goals. First, it finally granted the FDA power to order mandatory recalls of tainted food even when the farm or manufacturer resisted. Second, it required experts and industry to collaborate on writing guidelines for safe growing and handling of the 80 percent of foodstuffs covered by the FDA, then mandated all farms and facilities to have plans on file for following those guidelines. Next, it handed FDA jurisdiction over to the third-party auditors and assurance firms handling food imported into the United States—the federal government can now accredit third-party auditors in Mexico, or China, to a uniformly strict standard, and it can reject food from those who don't comply. (The FDA still can't tell domestic auditors what to do.[27] Optimists hope some of those accreditation standards will trickle over into domestic auditing, but the food industry will continue to resist the expense and the oversight.) Finally, the very existence of all these new rules implied a growth in FDA staff necessary to carry them out. The FDA might finally get more of the people it needed to raise the inspection standard that often fell below once every ten years to "never at all." After all, what good would it do for a future Jensen Farms to have a detailed food safety plan on file if no one ever went out to the farm and asked to see it? If there are no new boots on the ground, then what has really changed?

Food safety advocates hailed the changes as a fundamental shift of thinking toward attacking problems closer to their origins in the fields and packing sheds of American fruit and vegetable companies. Meat, poultry, pork, and most processed food inspections in the United States have traditionally focused on major production plants, whether slaughterhouses or factory-style produce or cooking operations—from the threshold to the shipping docks. The Food Safety Modernization Act's new produce standards would, in theory, enable the FDA to answer questions such as "What's happening back on the farm? What's the source of the contamination?" said Sandra Eskin, director of the Food Safety Campaign at the nonprofit The Pew Charitable Trusts.[28]

All the best-laid plans of a progressive government, though, run into the reality of congressional appropriations. In early 2012, the FDA presented a budget that included hundreds of millions of dollars in new spending to carry out both the demands of the act and new programs to improve the speed and safety of drug and medical device approvals. The Jensen Farms *Listeria* and thirty-three cantaloupe deaths were cited by name in the budget request as "the latest illustration of the continuing need for a strong food safety system."[29] Much of the increase was to come from new fees on food processors and handlers, rather than from general taxes. More and more of the FDA's budget in recent years has been sought through such user fees as a way of avoiding fights over limited pots of nondefense spending.[30]

But Congress still has to approve the user fees, and many Republicans don't like them. The fees are back-door tax increases, the thinking goes, eventually passed on to the consumer as higher prices. They force industry to pay for new regulations added to layers of rules they already find suffocating. So an expansion for the FDA was in doubt even before the "sequestration" battles at the end of 2012 put every government agency on hold. Deep, automatic budget cuts for all federal departments would hit by January 2013 unless a perpetually bickering Congress agreed on a comprehensive tax-and-spend plan. They hadn't managed to do that for years, in any long-term sense, instead passing a series of continuing resolutions that gave agencies no long-term direction. Like many other domestic agencies with powerful enemies—EPA, Interior, Education—each new budget of the FDA became a battleground of competing ideologies about what government should and shouldn't do. Hiring the hundreds and perhaps thousands of new FDA employees to carry out the food safety revolution was a long-term task. Congress for some time has rarely managed to look beyond its next recess.

Let's say for argument's sake the FDA in some magical year in the near future actually gets the modernization budget it asks for, and gets it in time to fill all the new positions before the next budget battle begins. How many people would that be? Remember, the FDA's oversight of 80 percent of the American food supply means responsibility for 350,000 food factories, warehouses, and farms. Then curb your enthusiasm with the number of new full-time domestic inspectors requested in the 2013 budget: exactly nineteen.[31] The FDA said those gains would be multiplied many times over by partnerships with state and local health agencies. Meanwhile, as Congress confronted plummeting revenue and entrenched budget battles from the 2008 recession onward, states and counties let go of 20 percent of their health departments' workforce. The recession's toll? A devastating attrition of more than thirty-four thousand health jobs.[32]

The deadly outbreaks and investigative scandals in popular foodstuffs such as cantaloupe, salad greens, peanuts, and eggs in the last decade took some of the public pressure off the meat and poultry industries. Their practices and the lack of preventive oversight from federal officials were thoroughly documented in state probes such as the Jack in the Box hamburger illnesses, and in populist exposes of high-calorie, high-fat culture such as Eric Schlosser's *Fast Food Nation* and the documentary *Food, Inc.* For all the spotlights trained on slaughterhouses during years of disturbing headlines about meat, from 2006 through 2011 U.S. consumers learned more about potential pathogens in previously innocuous foods such as melon and peanut butter.

Federal regulators in meat and poultry were not idle, however, while produce and processed foods caught the brunt of congressional scrutiny. Even as the FDA gained new power and sought bigger budgets, the USDA more quietly touted its own science-based revamping of safety practices for animal slaughter and packaging.

For decades the USDA system revolved around federal employees stationed permanently in slaughter plants, working with but not for the private companies packing beef and chicken. U.S. Food Safety and Inspection Service (FSIS) employees in poultry plants, for example, looked at every plucked chicken speeding by to warn of defects that could be signs of disease and contamination. In early 2012, the USDA said it wanted to go all-in with a new system developed in smaller pilot programs. The federal inspectors would no longer be responsible for approving every chicken. Instead, that job would fall back to the private company's employees, and the U.S. inspectors would concentrate on testing the chicken plant's safety systems and spot-checking for bacteria levels. The government said it would give private business back the job of pleasing the consumer with unblemished birds while saving federal spending for the job of guaranteeing safety.[33] Based on results from the pilot programs operating for years in some plants, the USDA said the changes could help prevent more than five thousand cases of *Salmonella* a year by zeroing in on the real hazards.[34]

But a coalition of consumer groups challenged the government's logic. The new system might save the USDA close to $100 million over three years, but wouldn't consumers want to know why? Because, critics said, the department would be cutting up to one thousand inspection jobs in the streamlined program. And how would it save the poultry industry hundreds of millions of dollars more? By speeding up the factory conveyors slinging chickens around the plants. The allowable speed under USDA rules was already 140 birds per minute. Now the government would let the lines speed up to 175 chickens every minute.[35] And only one employee had to be watching that line. That's three birds every second, passing by only one pair of eyeballs. A worker checks his watch for the next coffee break, and a dozen chicken carcasses have flown past unseen.

Federal regulators did move forward in recent years with safety measures for often-troubled ground beef products. The USDA's beef inspectors added six more strains of E. coli bacteria to the official list of "adulterants" in meat, meaning those batches of beef could not be shipped or sold if government or company tests came back positive. The department's Food Safety and Inspection Service also announced that it would implement a "test-and-hold" strategy for all ground beef that it was sampling for itself. That meant the batches of beef routinely sampled by FSIS-employed inspectors would not go out to the public until E. coli tests came back negative.

But as with most food initiatives challenged fiercely by industry, the two steps forward disguised lingering backwardness in the regulations. The "test and hold" applied only to those batches the FSIS swabbed, not to the batches the beef companies were testing for themselves. So tainted beef could go out the door and be subject to the chances of recall later on, after company tests showed up positive. And government inspectors generally uncovered the relentless creativity of industry in thwarting oversight. Slaughter employees told the inspectors in a 2012 report that one way they avoided hassles was to simply send off to the cooking department every single batch of beef the FSIS decided to test, without waiting to see if the test was positive.[36] A government policy said that if a positive batch was destroyed *or cooked*, the positive result would not count toward a threshold of samples after which the company had to take corrective actions. The government could turn up E. coli positive samples all week long, but as long as those random batches went to the industrial ovens to be precooked for lasagna or meatball customers, the slaughterhouse wouldn't have to own up to its basic problems with cleanliness on the cutting floor.

Two steps forward, one step back. Food safety groups sued the FDA in 2012 for missing multiple deadlines set in law by the 2011 modernization act. The FDA rebuffed them, told the courts that writing the rules was complicated, and finally started issuing the required rules months later. The new rules were scrupulously specific, down to how certain produce should be washed and loaded in coolers. Details on the rules in 2013 were accompanied by fierce warning letters from the FDA to farmers and packers, reminding them to brush up on the new safety details and get them right, for they would be inspected.[37] Cantaloupe growers got an admonition targeted straight at them, with the unusual warning that FDA inspectors would arrive at their doorstep precisely because the melons had become a national health problem.

But at the end of the same week, Congress and sequestration laid waste to the best-laid plans. The FDA, along with all other domestic agencies, took an 8 percent spending cut in every department, with little wiggle room on how to soften the blow on vital programs. Thousands of foreign and domestic inspections visits would be slashed, the agency said. And the news got worse farther down the food safety line. Not only would the FDA be in more danger of missing pathogens through fewer inspections, but the agencies responsible for tracking down pathogens once they got into the grocery stores would also face cuts. The CDC was set to lose $464 million in the first year of the automatic cuts. Some of that money would have paid for two thousand disease trackers, the ones the CDC hires directly or helps states and counties hire through grants. How soon would Americans notice the shrunken budget?, asked an editorialist at Nature.com, the weekly science magazine.[38]

This new "Starvation Diet," as they put it, "might not become apparent until the next time *Salmonella* poisons enter peanut butter."

3

TRACING TO SAFETY:
THE REAL LIFE "CSI" BEHIND
FOOD OUTBREAKS

When Colorado epidemiologist Alicia Cronquist learned two unrelated people were sick with *Listeria* bacteria at the same time, it was odd enough to make her take notice. What she didn't know yet, as those first cases trickled into the Colorado health department in late August 2011, was that she would have to help solve what would become the deadliest foodborne illness outbreak in modern American history.

Cronquist realized she was tracking an outbreak when two more reports of *Listeria*[1] poisoning arrived at the health department within a matter of days. Then two more the next day. And three the day after that. Whatever the contaminated food was, it was making a lot of people sick. Extremely sick. Among the first victims was an eighty-four-year-old man who thought he had a typical cold until he woke up shaking uncontrollably, and he was so ill he could not stand up.

It's the job of epidemiologists—detectives of the origin of disease—to pinpoint as quickly as possible which food is poisoning people. Much like crime sleuths hunting for a killer, they are racing to save lives. "Clearly, we were on high alert," said Cronquist, who was in charge of foodborne illness investigations for the Colorado Department of Public Health and Environment.

In a typical year, the state health department would see ten cases of *Listeria* reported by local labs and doctors' offices, who are required to tell public health officials whenever they confirm a case of *Listeria*, *Salmonella*, *E. coli*, and other key foodborne pathogens. In a typical August, state investigators would expect one case of *Listeria*. It was certainly odd, then, to see them coming in clusters of two or three patients at a time, within a matter of days of each other.

In Colorado that summer, Cronquist's suspicions launched several intense weeks of late-night brainstorming, blood samples rushed to the state lab, confiscations of half-eaten food from patients' refrigerators and, later, state scientists shopping for groceries and then swabbing them for contaminants. In the end, national officials would praise the state for record speed. Colorado's investigative work would lead hundreds of miles from Denver to a field of cantaloupe in Holly, a tiny farm town in the southeastern corner of the state.

Colorado ranks among the top states when it comes to foodborne illness detective work, and it is one of the CDC's go-to departments in terms of national surveillance. The state is one of ten chosen to participate in Food-Net, a federal program to monitor disease and link it to specific foods. Participation comes with extra federal cash for personnel and lab equipment, including the tools and training needed for DNA fingerprinting. State investigators track all foodborne infections in the Denver area by collecting lab reports, combing through hospital files, and interviewing patients about what they've eaten. The point of it all is to contribute to a national database that gauges the frequency of diseases and the culprit foods behind them.

Colorado became a "Food Center of Excellence" in 2012, one of five states researching the best ways to handle outbreak investigations. It's another federal designation that boosts the state's investigative power, although it doesn't come with funds to hire outbreak investigators. The likelihood that budgets for food safety investigation will expand is slim. Instead, cuts threaten to knock the level of safety down a notch. The head of the CDC, Dr. Tom Frieden, warned in 2013 that budget cuts are likely to result in lower funding for state teams on guard for patterns in foodborne illnesses, the first signs of outbreak. He predicted a loss of $300 million, not just for detective work in foodborne illness, but in preventing foreign diseases from entering and spreading through this country.[2]

The 2011 cantaloupe investigation was a model effort that might not have been solved as quickly in another state without Colorado's expertise. Unlike Colorado, some states do not have the capability to perform genetic tests that would match a *Listeria* strain found in contaminated food to an infection in a patient's body, for example. The massive, near-round-the-clock investigation began with questionnaires. State epidemiologists directed county health authorities to interview patients and their families, all using the same fifteen-page questionnaire Colorado uses when an outbreak is suspected. Each state has a preferred questionnaire to find out what food poisoning victims ate and where they bought it; the forms vary only slightly from one another. They are detailed, in depth, and memory jarring.

Did you eat at a cafeteria? Did you buy hummus? In the last four weeks, did you eat watermelon more than five times a week? The interviews are tedious and time-consuming for victims and their families. Sometimes, people get annoyed: How are they supposed to remember what they ate five weeks ago when they don't remember what they had for breakfast yesterday?

In the cantaloupe outbreak, the majority of victims were elderly, as they often are in foodborne illness outbreaks. The elderly, the young, and those with compromised immune systems are more susceptible to severe food poisoning. "The average age is in the 80s and they are quite ill," Cronquist said. "Their family members are at their bedside, and we are asking them to remember food that they ate a month ago. They are actually very difficult interviews."

At first, epidemiologists suspected the usual *Listeria* culprits—deli meats, hot dogs, dairy products. Several of the patients had eaten those foods. Scientists pulled some of them—along with whole and uncut cantaloupes—from refrigerators and brought them to the state food lab in Denver. Cantaloupe wasn't on the radar immediately; the 2011 outbreak was the first deadly one that would link *Listeria* with cantaloupe. Melon has a long, sordid history of causing sickness, but before 2011, cantaloupe was nearly always linked to *Salmonella*.

As one set of health authorities was questioning patients, another group was collecting blood samples and isolating the *Listeria* bacteria. Those samples, called "isolates," went to the state lab in a brick building on the east side of Denver. There, state microbiologist Hugh Maguire's team deconstructed the DNA profiles in the bacteria to see if the patients had the same strain.

The DNA profiles are uploaded to a national database kept by the Centers for Disease Control and Prevention. The database—called PulseNet—is a key investigative tool that federal officials say has significantly cut the amount of time it takes to find the source of an outbreak. In rapid time, federal epidemiologists at the CDC in Atlanta can see whether the same strain of bacteria sickening people in Colorado is wreaking havoc elsewhere.

In the cantaloupe outbreak of 2011, more than one strain was identified, and those strains were not just sickening and killing people in Colorado, but Nebraska, Texas, and New Mexico, among many others. The outbreak would eventually spread to twenty-eight states.[3]

Within five days of suspecting an outbreak, the Colorado state lab had determined that two patients had matching strains, and another two patients had a different matching strain. Already, there were two separate strains identified within the outbreak. With hundreds of strains of *Listeria*, two or more can sit side by side on the same food. The fact that scientists were now tracking two did not necessarily mean there were two sources. "It just means we have a deeper mystery," Cronquist said. In the end, five different strains were linked to the same cantaloupe farm.

Epidemiologists in the counties where the patients lived set out for another round of interviews. One epidemiologist interviewed two patients with the same strain of *Listeria* to listen better for common patterns; another interviewed the other matched pair.

That same day, the state health department sent out a *Listeria* alert by fax and email to doctors, emergency rooms, hospitals, and labs. And the public received the first notice of an outbreak, a warning for those susceptible to the illness—the elderly, the pregnant, and those with compromised immune systems—to avoid deli meats and unpasteurized cheese. Cantaloupe was not mentioned. The health emergency was dire enough that state health officials needed to warn the public, but they didn't know yet what to warn them about. They were guessing. "We were telling people not to eat deli meats. We had no concrete message to give," Cronquist said.

The public health warning with a vaguely mentioned culprit—maybe cheese, maybe meat—was a rare move. Colorado issues, on average, only one public warning per year regarding an outbreak. The state health department puts out an average of thirty-three notices per year warning the public of food that has been recalled, from peanut butter to crackers to ground beef. The recalls most often come before there has ever been a report of anyone ill. They are typically the result of routine testing at production plants, and reasons vary from pathogen contamination to mislabeling to bits of metal or plastic that inadvertently fell into the food.[4]

It would take one more week for Colorado officials to tell the public it was cantaloupe that was making people deathly sick. Epidemiologists at the state lab were beginning to zero in on melon. Cantaloupe is on the patient questionnaire, but not emphasized. At first, the fact that several patients had eaten cantaloupe didn't stand out. After all, the melon hadn't been linked to a *Listeria* outbreak before, and it was August, the peak of the melon season in Colorado, so the fact that people were eating it wasn't unusual.

Cronquist turned to the CDC database created by the FoodNet survey, the nation's most accurate gauge on what the general population is eating. It's where epidemiologists go to check the baseline for healthy people. How likely is it, for example, for an American to eat sushi on any given day? Certainly a lower percentage than eating at McDonald's, but if half of the people who got sick in one outbreak had eaten tuna sushi, a Japanese restaurant is likely where investigators would look first. Or, if epidemiologists were tracking a summer outbreak on the West Coast among people who reported eating salsa, they might query the database to find out how common it is that West Coasters in general eat tomatoes in July. How likely are American women to eat spinach on a weekly basis? Or peanut butter on toast? The database is maintained by the CDC's enteric disease epidemiology branch, which surveys people in different regions of the country aiming to capture America's diverse eating habits. When national investigators are tracking an outbreak, the FoodNet team can answer a query within a matter of hours.

As useful as the database can be, however, it is badly out of date; the last eating surveillance took place in the early 2000s. Imports of seafood and other suspect foods have risen sharply since then, while food processing techniques also have changed dramatically. Eating habits evolve quickly in this country. Grocery stores didn't routinely offer Mediterranean olive bars and sushi trays back in 2002, for example. The survey is expensive, and there hasn't been money in the budget to keep it up to date.

In Colorado that summer of 2011, Alicia Cronquist wanted to know how likely it was for *Listeria* victims to eat cantaloupe. The answer from FoodNet was 65 percent. There was her "aha" moment. Of the patients Cronquist had been tracking, 100 percent reported eating cantaloupe. And Cronquist knew one of them still had it in the refrigerator.

The patient had purchased two melons, cutting one into pieces and putting it in the refrigerator. The second cantaloupe was still whole. State investigators gathered those cantaloupes and brought them to the lab for testing. Meanwhile, two state employees went grocery shopping around metro Denver, buying fifteen cantaloupes. They tested the rind, as well as the flesh of the melons, for *Listeria* bacteria.

The lab work was rushed. If protocol was to incubate the swabs of the cantaloupe for four to sixteen hours, scientists incubated the specimens for "four hours on the dot," Maguire said.[5] His lab fast-tracked the genetic matching to find out whether the bacteria strains from patients' blood samples matched the strains in the melon. To finish the work as fast as possible, the lab set aside routine lab work, such as tests that make sure milk is properly pasteurized, or others that track bacteria count on raw meat.

Five cantaloupes from one store tested negative for *Listeria*. But all ten melons from the other store were contaminated with the bacteria. What's more, the strains of *Listeria* found on those ten melons matched strains found in the ill patients. "Everything we were seeing in the patients, we were seeing in the cantaloupe," Maguire said.

One week after the first public warning, health authorities announced they had linked the source of the poisoning to cantaloupe. The cheese, deli meats, and dairy industries were in the clear this time, and while those officials exhaled in relief, the produce industry braced for the onslaught of attention—the bad kind.

As more patient blood samples arrived at the state lab, they fell into three distinct strains, their DNA pattern matching side by side on a state computer screen like barcodes from a grocery store. Cantaloupe taken from patient refrigerators—both cut and uncut—had the same strains. But the confiscated cantaloupe did not have a sticker naming the farm.

In interviews, though, patients were saying they had eaten cantaloupe from Colorado's most well-known melon-growing region, a town called Rocky Ford. "Patients were spontaneously telling us the cantaloupe said 'Rocky Ford' on it," Cronquist said. "That was coming out loud and clear. Some patients called it 'extra sweet,' which we all know is why it is so delicious."

The CDC refined its public health warning, this time not just naming cantaloupe, but specifically melon from the renowned Rocky Ford area of southeastern Colorado. It was a warning that would cause backlash from Rocky Ford's farmers, who suffered as cantaloupe consumption dropped after the scare—up to an 80 percent drop, according to national estimates. Rocky Ford farmers claimed their reputation was tarnished unfairly, especially since the cantaloupe was later linked to a farm in Holly, some ninety miles away from Rocky Ford. The farm at fault—Jensen Farms—had borrowed the famed Rocky Ford name on its cantaloupe for marketing purposes.

As the food tracking continued, investigators knocked on the door of Herb Stevens, the eighty-four-year-old patient who woke up shaking uncontrollably, had a fever of 102.7, and couldn't stand up. Stevens lay seriously ill in a hospital bed in the Denver suburb of Littleton. Investigators wanted to talk to his wife, eighty-one-year-old Elaine. What did she serve to eat over the last month? Elaine couldn't recall all of that, but she had something better than her memory: all of her King Soopers credit card receipts. She saved them to make sure she got all the frequent flier miles she earned by using her credit card. Health officials were also able to get her loyalty card information for the grocery store, so they could check her purchases and see for themselves exactly what the Stevenses had been eating.[6]

Grocery store records gathered from patients showed which cantaloupe they purchased and on what days. Then, the FDA was able to track the melon purchases back to the distribution trucks, then back to the farm. The FDA narrowed the focus of the investigation to two farms, including Jensen Farms near Holly. Federal investigators descended on the farm, taking samples from soil and machinery.

Just two days passed between the state health department's warning to avoid Rocky Ford cantaloupe and a new warning. They had pinpointed the farm. Jensen Farms recalled the killer melons on September 14, 2011, about two weeks after the first reports of sick people began surfacing.

The next morning, Colorado grocery stores launched automated tools to spread more warnings about cantaloupe. King Soopers has the phone numbers of loyalty card customers, and the store scanners recognize whether they bought cantaloupe. Upon news of the recall, grocery officials pushed the button on a robocall system that contacted each cantaloupe consumer and urged them to heed the recall. Among those who received a robocall was the Stevenses' daughter, Jeni Exley. She, too, had bought a cantaloupe from the contaminated farm back in August. The melon never made Jeni sick, but the one her dad had eaten had thrown the family's lives into turmoil.

Herb Stevens was so ill from the cantaloupe he had to move into a nursing home. He never rebounded, never regained the strength to garden or walk without help. He died in July 2013.

Laura Gieraltowski, an epidemiologist on the CDC's foodborne outbreak investigation team in Atlanta, thinks of herself as a detective of sorts. Each week, she tracks up to twenty or thirty "clusters"—groups of people across the nation with the same strain of bacteria making them sick, more people than what epidemiologists would normally expect. Foodborne illness bacteria collected from patient blood samples is uploaded to the CDC's PulseNet, which spits out periodic reports for Gieraltowski and her teammates.[7] Many of the clusters fade out soon after they are noticed, without public warning or a product recall. That wasn't the case with a cluster of patients, mostly children, who were showing up in doctor offices and hospitals across the country with matching strains of *Salmonella bredeney* in the fall of 2012.

Gieraltowski was the lead investigator on that outbreak, which began, as usual, mysteriously. The early reports were that many of the sick children's families shopped at Trader Joe's, and based on interviews, these kids weren't eating the standard American kid fare of frozen chicken nuggets and macaroni and cheese. They were eating organic snacks and drinking soy and almond milk.

She held conference calls with local investigators in the twenty states where kids were sick, stricken with fever, diarrhea, and stomach cramps. The brainstorming first focused on milk and eventually wound around to organic peanut butter. Almost every family had shopped at Trader Joe's, but only 60 percent of them remembered buying and eating peanut butter. Among those who reported eating peanut butter, though, several recalled the particular kind of peanut butter: Trader Joe's Valencia. "That was the red flag," Gieraltowski recalled.

She wasn't deterred by the fact that not everyone recalled eating that particular peanut butter, or any peanut butter at all. Rarely do 100 percent of people report eating the contaminated food that made them all sick. "Most people have trouble remembering what they ate yesterday," Gieraltowski said, and it takes two or three weeks for *Salmonella* infections to make people sick enough to seek medical treatment. Plus, this was a case involving kids. "Maybe they ate a Trader Joe's peanut butter sandwich at a friend's house. Maybe you interview the mom but the mom doesn't know what the dad gave them," she said.

A few of the states were able to collect some of the peanut butter from the pantries of sick children. In Washington, lab tests matched the strain found in the peanut butter to the blood samples collected from patients. Almost immediately after hearing the brand name—Valencia—CDC investigators notified the FDA so trackers there could begin finding out which plant makes Valencia. The search would lead them to Sunland, Inc., in Portales, New Mexico.[8]

Sunland recalled hundreds of products, including peanut butter, almond butter, and cashew butter. The FDA confiscated peanut butter from the Sunland nut butter plant and found the same strain of *Salmonella bredeney*.

Among the forty-two people reported ill, the average age was seven. Ten of those victims were hospitalized. No one died, perhaps in part because of the detective work that led Gieraltowski and her team to the source of the outbreak within several days. Gieraltowski calls it "shoe leather epidemiology." Evolving technology—databases including PulseNet and FoodNet and computer records like grocery store frequent shopper cards—speeds investigative work, but much of it still happens in interviews with patients and brainstorming sessions among epidemiologists that connect the dots. Those skills are evolving with the ever-changing American food chain. They've learned to ask more complex questions. "It's just on the radar to ask, 'What spices do you use when you cook?'" Gieraltowski said. At first, it might seem it's the salami that's sickening people, but on closer look, it's the peppers inside the salami.

It was after the Sunland peanut butter scare that the FDA for the first time used its new enforcement authority to halt operations at a food plant. The federal agency suspended production at the country's largest organic peanut butter processor on powers gained through the 2011 Food Safety Modernization Act. The law gives the FDA authority to intercede on company operations when there is "reasonable probability" of causing serious health problems or death, an action that prior to the 2011 law would have required the FDA to seek court action.[9] The plant reached a deal with federal authorities to reopen about a month after the forced shutdown. Included in the deal was a requirement that Sunland hire an independent expert to develop a sanitation plan.[10]

The 2012 peanut butter outbreak, like the 2011 *Listeria* outbreak, ended with fingers pointed directly at the source of the problem. But that's not always how it goes. Sometimes, foodborne illness investigators know exactly which manufacturer or food store chain shipped the contaminated food to grocery stores or handed it through the window in the drive-thru lane, yet they don't tell us.

The federal government's tendency to avoid naming names, safe food advocates say, robs consumers of vital information. In an October 2011 *Salmonella* outbreak that sickened sixty-eight, federal agencies told journalists there was no public benefit in being more specific than problems at "Restaurant Chain A."

It was the Oklahoma health department that disclosed the chain where many victims had eaten was Taco Bell, but not because it had planned on telling the public. Taco Bell's identity was revealed after journalists from *Food Safety News* and other outlets filed a public information request with the state health department in Oklahoma, one of several states where people were getting sick after eating fast-food tacos.[11] The reporters wanted documents related to the outbreak investigation. Oklahoma health officials released them without redacting the restaurant name.

The CDC's final report on the outbreak, which spread across ten states, still identifies the source as "Restaurant Chain A."[12]

The Oklahoma State Department of Health had not previously revealed Taco Bell's name in any press release that warned of the outbreak. Their reason? By the time health officials figured out what was causing the illnesses, the threat had passed. The cluster of people who were ill was no longer growing. Also, food investigators were never able to pinpoint the exact ingredient that was contaminated, although 90 percent of the ill reported they ate lettuce. "If there is no ongoing threat, a decision might be made to not put out any public notification at that time," said Lawrence Burnsed, director of the Oklahoma department's communicable disease division.[13]

Several other state health departments around the country cited confidentiality in denying the records requests.

National epidemiologists all but ruled out ground beef, even though 94 percent of people reported their Taco Bell meal contained beef. The way "Restaurant Chain A" handles and cooks its beef gave them little reason to suspect the meat. Also, the epidemic curve of the outbreak—a sharp increase and decline in victims that lasted one or two months—gave the impression the bad food was produce, not meat.

The FDA could not crack the case, despite trying to track back from the restaurants to delivery trucks to the suppliers. The agency analyzed the supply truck delivery routes and schedules to various Taco Bells, trying to create a timeline or connection between food deliveries and Taco Bell customers who grew sick. Investigators discovered that the onset of customers' illnesses was linked to more than one food shipment—not helpful in trying to nail the precise food and farm.

Even though federal investigators could not for certain say the Salmonella-tinged food was in fact lettuce, or cheese or tomatoes, and even though it seemed that whatever had made people sick was gone from the food chain, many health advocates criticized the CDC for not naming Taco Bell. Didn't consumers have a right to know, they asked, that Taco Bell was serving food that sent people to emergency rooms with abdominal cramps and bloody diarrhea, forcing them to miss work or school for several days? Shouldn't consumers have that knowledge to use as they see fit—whether it's to avoid Taco Bell, or to figure it could have happened at any restaurant and carry on eating there?

For some, it was especially troubling that the federal government was protecting Taco Bell when it wasn't the first time in recent years the Mexican fast-food chain was linked to a national outbreak.

Just a year prior, in the summer of 2010, 155 people in twenty-one states were sickened by Salmonella in an outbreak linked to Taco Bell restaurants, according to Oklahoma public health records.[14] Following the same protocol as in 2011, the CDC's final report again refers to the source of the contaminated food as "Restaurant Chain A" and not Taco Bell. And same as in 2011, epidemiologists were not able to pinpoint which Taco Bell ingredient was tainted.

The FDA, in response to harsh criticism for not revealing Taco Bell's name in 2011, issued this statement:

FDA strives to provide reliable information and be as transparent and proactive as possible, particularly when there is an issue that threatens the public health. In situations where there are current illnesses associated with a specific food manufactured by a specific firm, or contaminated foods are distributed without known illnesses, FDA will continue to issue health advisories and press releases, as needed, to provide consumers with specific information so they may take steps to decrease their risk of illness and avoid further exposures.

We will also continue to work with CDC and State health officials to provide support during their investigations. We are currently re-examining our practices and policies to ensure they will provide as much transparency as possible while adhering to laws and regulations.

The CDC stuck with "Restaurant Chain A" for its final report on the outbreak, despite that Oklahoma had disclosed many of the victims had eaten at Taco Bell. In a statement, Taco Bell said the CDC had never discovered the definitive source, but they acknowledged that some of the victims had eaten at the chain.[15]

Kansas State's Powell argued for more disclosure. At the least, he said, CDC policy should make it clear why the agency names some restaurants and producers and not others. "If Taco Bell keeps making people sick with lettuce, I want to know it's Taco Bell," he said. "How bright are they in choosing their lettuce suppliers?"[16]

Cronquist said Colorado tries to strike a balance. If the public is still at risk from food, companies are identified. But the state also needs compliance from various facilities while it investigates. Moreover, victim interviews can be skewed by early disclosure; if they have heard "Taco Bell" or "green onions," it can bias their answers.

Perhaps worse than not naming names is a failure by the FDA to pursue certain national outbreaks—especially those involving leafy green vegetables. Foodborne illness investigators in some states call it the federal government's "cone of silence"; a problem because investigators at the state level have to rely on federal agencies when outbreaks cross state lines.

One such case began in the summer of 2009. In Colorado, it was state fair time, a time of year that always causes anxiety among foodborne illness officials. The crowds, heat, open-air food booths, portable trailers serving up tacos and chili cheese fries. It's like asking for trouble. When the state lab connected two cases in children of the sometimes deadly *E. coli* O157:H7 by matching their DNA strains, investigators acted quickly.

Both kids had gone to the Colorado State Fair, investigators from two counties learned through patient questionnaires. State officials urged them to go back to the families with more questions and try to nail down where exactly the kids ate, and what foods.

As they waited for more answers, researchers in Minnesota, Iowa, and three other states loaded illness cases into the national network that tracks DNA fingerprints of food-illness bacteria strains. Ill people in Minnesota, Iowa, and North Carolina had eaten at the same Italian-style restaurant in Omaha, Nebraska, in early September. When Colorado got its deeper case histories back, it found both state victims had eaten at an Italian-style restaurant in Pueblo. It wasn't the state fair connection, after all.

More questions zeroed in on house salads. Even when the victims hadn't ordered salad, they had nibbled from a family member's plate. Eight of ten cases had eaten lettuce at a restaurant, according to a Colorado outbreak memo obtained through the open records act. States tried to find out the restaurants' suppliers. Colorado learned that the lettuce used in Pueblo came from a major produce supplier in the Salinas Valley of California, Tanimura and Antle, which did not respond to requests for comment.

The patients, meanwhile, made slow recoveries. Some were in the hospital for days. *E. coli* is particularly worrisome to food experts because it can cause severe gastroenteritis, pneumonia, and kidney failure.

And then the FDA and CDC dropped the case.

"I will forever be mad that the FDA didn't pursue" those 2009 *E. coli* cases, said Kirk Smith, a veterinarian and supervisor of the foodborne disease investigation section of the Minnesota Department of Health. "It was a smaller outbreak, but still, if you figure out what the food is, even after the fact, you can hopefully get back to where that food was produced and perhaps correct something so there's not a bigger outbreak in the future."[17]

Public health officials in Colorado and Minnesota privately vented frustration and derision at the FDA for going easy on food producers through "hypocritical" silence, and for failing to pluck the "low-hanging fruit" of pathogen knowledge available in an outbreak probe. Instead of tracing the cases back to the farm and figuring out how a potentially deadly bacteria was making its way onto lettuce, the cases stayed in food safety's bureaucratic background.

The FDA's decision to let the six-state *E. coli* probe go dormant, despite clear leads, blocked efforts to force better growing and packing methods. "As someone who is out in fields with farmers, it's really hard to get them excited about food safety if they never hear about other outbreaks," said Doug Powell, a Kansas State University food scientist who advocates for wider probes and public disclosure. "We have evidence that telling stories makes a difference."

State-level investigators realized the federal government was dropping the case when they asked for a status update on the probe. According to email records released to the *Denver Post* under open records laws, CDC epidemiologist Colin Schwensohn told the states "with no recent cases, this cluster is less of a priority." The threat had passed, so the federal agencies would not pursue the cause.

Minnesota's Smith fired back: "I think it is a huge mistake for FDA to drop this." Smith's email to the CDC and other investigators, which he acknowledged was a "rant," went on: "If FDA won't fully engage and work backwards from two restaurants on a rock solid lead, then all of their claims about making things better are all so much talk."

Colorado officials were also irritated. "Colorado and other states challenged this decision, but FDA did not change its position about pursuing the traceback further," according to a state memo. Colorado epidemiologist Alicia Cronquist said in an interview, "We were extremely frustrated." State investigators voiced their complaints in a conference call with federal officials, arguing a deeper probe could help prevent future outbreaks.

The FDA declined comment, beyond the limited information about the federal agencies' reasoning contained in emails at the time. Neither the FDA nor the CDC offered responses to specific questions about the 2009 outbreak, or to general questions about how investigations end.

The case may have been weakened by lack of a key lab link. Investigators prefer to have positive tests for pathogens on the food itself, matching results from patients. In the 2009 outbreak, the suspect food was long gone. Colorado officials acknowledged the failure to follow through on the investigation was related to money. "We all operate under pretty severe financial restraints, and we need to pick and choose which clusters we investigate, and which tracebacks are performed," Cronquist said.

The unsatisfying conclusion to the 2009 *E. coli* cases bothered some food experts, beyond the failure to put "boots on the farm" and search for pathogens. They also wanted state and federal officials to name names more often and to put pressure on businesses by exposing those who fail.

"Consumers of food have a right to know, period. And as taxpayers, consumers have a right to know what public health officials know about those same food producers," said Seattle attorney Bill Marler, one of the nation's top foodborne illness litigators.

Early emails in the 2009 outbreak identified the restaurants that consumers said they had in common. Colorado named the produce grower, Tanimura and Antle, in its wrap-up memo, but said the restaurants did not appear to be at fault. Tanimura and Antle did not return calls seeking comment.

Despite their other frustrations, some public health officials say the FDA is making progress in outbreak investigations overall. They say the agency has streamlined its outbreak teams and can move quickly, as evidenced by rapid conclusions in the Colorado cantaloupe probe. Minnesota's Smith said his 2009 "rant" was "the nadir of working with the FDA. Since then, in part we hope because of our harping, they know they need to do more. Things aren't perfect, but they are still progressing."

4

THE WHOLE WORLD
IN YOUR KITCHEN

It's late on a Saturday afternoon in the backyard, the smoke from the grill is drifting off in a breeze, blowing across a picnic table piled with fresh summer fruit, overflowing salad bowls, and platters layered with spicy cheeses, olives, and shrimp cocktail. The bounty of fun food is the backdrop to an all-American day.

Except that, more likely than not, much of the food on the burdened picnic table isn't "American" at all.

Those hamburgers are a don't-ask-don't-tell compilation of beef leftovers shaved from higher-quality cuts of meat in slaughterhouses ranging from Uruguay to Canada. By the time those beef patties arrive at the grocery store, they may each include bits and pieces of a couple of foreign nations, not to mention a half-dozen U.S. states.

The strawberries in the salad bowl may have come from as far away as Chile, conditions unknown, or from farm fields of dubious operators in Mexico where produce furrows float on rivers of garbage-strewn irrigation waters. The pineapples hail from Thailand, the clementines from Spain, the grapes from any number of Latin American exporters.[1]

The shrimp on the cocktail platter may trace back to volatile Gulf of Mexico waters made alternately famous and infamous by New Orleans chefs and contaminated seafood beds. But much of the shrimp consumed by Americans is now grown at aquatic farms in China and other cheap-labor nations of Asia.

If the cheese selections include queso fresco, then that unpasteurized delicacy hails from proud and sometimes risky cultural traditions in Mexico.

Scattered throughout and sprinkled on top of anything from the picnic hummus bowl to the varietal olive snacks are spices ranging from Santo Domingo hot peppers to Sri Lankan cardamom.

Contamination from every one of those foods has government inspectors and university food safety experts worrying about imports more and more each year.

The Centers for Disease Control and Prevention in 2012 released a five-year study of foodborne illness outbreaks from imported goods, and they found statistics heading in a troubling direction. Fifteen different nations sent food to the United States that resulted in outbreaks of pathogens, with the rate increasing markedly in the last two years of the study.[2] The thirty-nine foreign-food outbreaks caused 2,348 illnesses, with nearly half of implicated food coming from Asian shippers. Pathogens in fish caused the largest number of import-related outbreaks, with the next largest group caused by various spices.

The pressure of massive imported food volume pressing against the tenuous FDA and USDA inspection screens is relentless, and growing. A surprisingly self-critical report from the FDA in 2011 detailed the rising wave: 80 percent of the seafood consumed in America was already coming from imports.[3] Americans want strawberries in January, oranges in November, and bananas all year long—in certain seasons, 60 percent of the produce being sold in U.S. grocery stores comes from farms abroad. All told, up to 15 percent of all the food eaten in America is coming from overseas imports, and that will accelerate. The FDA report put future growth at about 15 percent per year. We want those strawberries, but we also demand they come cheap, as the power of consumer choice goads giant retailers such as Walmart, Costco, and Safeway into ruthless negotiations with suppliers to provide cut-rate goods. "The manufacturers and producers that FDA regulates face intense pressure to lower costs and improve productivity," the agency said.[4]

Food, drugs, medical devices, and other imported items regulated by the FDA are referred to in port-of-entry business lingo as "lines"—crates of pineapples from a ship are one "line" of goods on a customs and inspection invoice, while frozen shrimp from the adjacent cargo hold constitute another "line." A food industry consultant and former FDA official estimated the number of imported "lines" the agency sees coming in each year have shot from about five million a few years ago to more than thirty million.[5]

This extension of the U.S. food pipeline around the world has often occurred well out of sight and certainly out of mind for the American consumer. We call for instant availability of anything we might want to eat, and overwhelming choice, without thinking there might not be quite enough apple trees in Washington state to satisfy our craving for apple juice at a hotel buffet in early March. Food toxicologist Robert Buchanan, head of the University of Maryland's food safety program, likes to quiz people from outside his trade exactly where they think their chosen meal originated.

The number one producer of apple juice is China, he noted, followed by Chile and then Germany.[6] Orange juice, though, must be an all-American item, what with those friendly commercials from Florida growers in overalls and the abundance of trees in the citrus belt, right? The number one producer of orange juice is Brazil, Buchanan demurs, providing nearly half of the billion liters of orange juice imported into the United States each year. A brief panic over a banned fungicide found on Brazilian oranges sent juice futures spiking and had regulators scrambling to rethink their system in early 2012—U.S. food safety officials found traces of a mold inhibitor barred on U.S. farms but allowed in Brazil.[7]

Think about it another way, Buchanan suggested, with the help of any household globe. If you want to know where your food is coming from, just put a finger on the tip of South America at the beginning of the southern summer in December, then trace northward at two-week intervals as the prime growing season follows the sun. By the time you've hit Alaska, you've covered half the globe, and farmers and distributors operating under a near-infinite variety of food safety conditions.

How many inspectors does the FDA have to look at those millions of wildly disparate, highly perishable items arriving at U.S. ports? About 1,800, with constant calls for federal spending freezes threatening even that stretched level of coverage. That translates, according to the government's own numbers, to less than 2 percent of imported food actually getting inspected each year.[8]

The conditions at the other end of the import pipeline, meanwhile, range from the reassuring to the deeply disturbing.

Major produce growers adopting the best of U.S. food safety standards after decades of trial and error are opening new farms and packing centers in Mexico, which draw on deep well water cleaner than some American supplies.

But there are horrific scenes in plain sight at other foreign packers. Bloomberg reporters visited a Mexican grape tomato farm and saw clouds of fecal dust blowing from latrines over the fields.[9] Workers had no place to wash their hands after relieving themselves. University of Georgia food safety researcher Michael Doyle describes farms relying on garbage-strewn irrigation water that flowed through Mexico City before offering dubious nourishment to plantations growing export crops.[10]

The pressures on seafood farming operations are new and growing, as natural ocean supplies get fished out at the same time a rising consumer class in developing nations finds money for new sources of protein to add to their traditional diets. Anybody who has ever dangled a marshmallow or a cheeseball on the end of a line and watched perch, bass, and crawfish rush up for a bite has an instinctive sense of just how much a remote seafood farm could get away with in fattening up fish. Fish farm culture lends itself to a "garbage in, who-knows-what-out" mentality, as aquatic creatures convert nearly any form of edible substance to valuable flesh. The same group of Bloomberg reporters went in search of trouble at fish farms in China and Vietnam, where laborers strive to meet enormous worldwide demand for shrimp and once-exotic tilapia. The Chinese tilapia farm fattened tilapia for the U.S. market with shovels full of pig and geese feces.[11] Researchers say *Salmonella* clings to much of the revolting feed. At Vietnamese shrimp packers, reporters found companies packing the seafood in local tap water that health authorities say should be boiled for purity before human use. Those shrimp are potentially floating in all sorts of bacteria for the days-long trip in a cargo hold to a U.S. port.

Asked what imported seafood he's willing to venture, Georgia's Doyle quickly responded with a geographic checklist. "You don't buy shrimp or tilapia from Asia. Most is coming from China, and the conditions that much of it is grown in are not what we would consider to be equivalent to the sanitary standards and practices of the U.S.," Doyle said. "I like shrimp. But we buy it from the Gulf of Mexico."[12]

The Chinese melamine scandals alerted U.S. regulators and consumers to a threat even more terrifying than the dangers of stray bacteria. How can the import system possibly screen out food intentionally doctored in other nations for greater profits, in a complex supply chain that ranges from multinational dairies down to struggling family farmers?

The melamine horror unfolded slowly in 2008, yet it reached such enormous proportions through China's outsized population that the rest of the world couldn't help but pay attention.[13] Babies raised on China's cheap powdered-milk infant formulas went into kidney failure and developed deeply painful kidney stones. Reports of illnesses and warnings of suspect formula had been trickling in for months; with an eye toward the Chinese government's history of censorship, media outlets theorized the scarier details were being suppressed by authorities trying to minimize the damage during the publicity blitz surrounding the 2008 Beijing Olympics.[14] Yet this story was simply too big to control, with three hundred thousand babies eventually making the official victim tallies. At least six of them died, and hundreds were hospitalized. Multiple dairies were implicated, and investigations revealed disturbingly systemic holes in China's safety net, rather than a more reassuring focus on one source that could quickly be cleaned up.[15] Farmers and middlemen throughout Chinese milk production stretched dairy supplies by adding water to raw milk, then bought various supplements that could boost the milk's protein content back to an acceptable level for sale. One of the widely available supplements was melamine, a chemical used primarily for manufacturing flame-resistant plastics. Perhaps it goes without saying that most chemicals that could, say, protect an overworked automobile oil filter from bursting into flames are not likely safe inside the human stomach. Some farmers and producers appeared to know what they were dumping into milk, while others blindly bought supplements touted as safe, soy-based additives.

U.S. consumers largely escaped any of the danger, as dairy producers and formula makers here have until recently relied on a more local supply. Yet ripples of the scandal reflected the growing complexity of global markets— a popular Asian chew candy called White Rabbit was widely available at Chinese grocery stores in the West, and many households bought it as an intriguing novelty. Connecticut authorities, among others, found melamine in the candies, and recalls ensued.[16]

The government reaction in China was that paradox of the lingering powers of dictatorship: the same officials who could so blithely cover up a scandal with delay and censorship could also crack down mercilessly on the spotlighted offenders once the public knew enough to demand punishment. In the United States, food safety advocates wait for years after the fact to learn if food executives clearly involved in scandals will ever be prosecuted, from scandals resulting in far more deaths than the Chinese melamine incidents. Those advocates say they would even feel some vindication from the minor relief of a misdemeanor charge or two so long as those responsible at a farm or warehouse accepted blame, by name, for contaminated food. In China, meanwhile, prosecution, when it came, was swift and brutal. Two people accused of misusing the toxic materials to stretch milk were executed.[17] Other dairy and supply executives got dozens of years in jail, while provincial government leaders resigned under fire.

The tainted milk and powder hardened international assumptions about China's opaque and possibly dangerous food supply. The 2008 milk scandal was preceded by an international melamine scare in pet food, with hundreds and perhaps thousands of U.S. pets dying of kidney complications.[18] The pet food worries spread into the human food chain, as the FDA and USDA ran tests to reassure consumers after the same melamine-tainted vegetable protein was found in the feed of chickens and pigs sold for human consumption. And the 2008 milk scandal was followed by more of the same. Despite assurances of radical overhauls to Chinese food oversight, large amounts of melamine-saturated dairy products were found at major dairies again in 2009 and 2010.[19]

The vast scale of the melamine problems seemed to unnerve many U.S. food safety officials. It's one thing to combat spot contaminations caused by stubborn environmental pathogens. Produce and animals are raised in and on dirt, after all, and innovative scientists can always find more ways to try to scrub them clean of accidental threats. But to combat intentional contamination prompted by systemic economic pressures, in a hugely influential nation halfway around the world—that seemed a far more impossible task. Exports from China will grow 426 percent from 2009 to 2020, the FDA said in a report on international food safety challenges, and will then constitute nearly 20 percent of all foreign trade around the world.[20] And the nature of the food in question didn't help calm inspectors' nerves. Milk powder winds up in everything from infant formula to protein-rich power bars. How could those overburdened U.S. port inspectors possibly hope to keep up? University researchers finally shrug their shoulders in dismay and say what diplomatic FDA and USDA bureaucrats won't: "There are some countries that just aren't ethical," a microbiologist said.

China appeared to make some headway with U.S. regulators and consumers in 2013, finally winning approval to export poultry products to America after years of worries about avian flu strains and other food safety questions. But reading between the lines of the announcement would give most poultry consumers pause—China can only send the U.S. cooked chicken, and the bird parts can't be Chinese.[21] They must be U.S. chickens exported to China, processed, and then sent back, or birds that China imports from another country already approved for exporting chickens directly to U.S. markets. Not exactly a full-fledged endorsement.

The FDA itself says in recent budget documents that the rapid advancement of foreign foods into the average U.S. consumer diet means there is no longer any distinction, from a food safety inspector's point of view, between imported and domestic goods. The agency had long counted on new authority in the 2011 Food Safety Modernization Act to overhaul its screening of food imports. In 2013, the agency boasted of opening liaison offices in the largest countries exporting food to America, while pressing for more inspection powers inside foreign food distributors. Reality set in when congressional budget fights guaranteed FDA budget cuts instead of the steep increases food safety officials said they needed to carry out mandates in the act. Given the agency's thin and increasingly strained resources, the honest assessment of imports can be read another way: imported foods will be inspected just like domestic foods, which is to say, almost never.

The 2011 act, which even skeptical consumer groups agree is the most important leap forward in food safety laws in America in eighty years, theoretically gives the FDA new powers in the following ways:

1. The United States can demand that third-party auditors checking overseas food companies—those self-interested foxes also guarding the hen houses of domestic food production—must meet certain uniform standards for auditing and receive official certification.[22] In other words, an audit of the auditors, with the force of U.S. government approval and denial behind the reviews. It should be noted Congress was very careful to allow such oversight only with importers. There is no plan to demand certification of domestic third-party auditors, despite their apparently overlooking so many warning signs in the peanut fiasco, and the egg debacle, and the cantaloupe *Listeria* disaster. The FDA can't do anything about those auditors charged with assessing the food safety of farms and companies on U.S. soil.

2. The FDA will put more "boots on the ground" in foreign nations, expanding its system of overseas offices with inspectors intent on checking the operations of major food exporters in Beijing, Mumbai, northern Mexico, and dozens more potential locales. The law demands the FDA double the number of inspections of overseas food facilities every year for the first five years of the act.[23]

3. Foreign food growers, distributors, manufacturers, and exporters now have the burden of proving their food is safe. Amazingly, this basic, assumptive tenet did not have the force of law before the 2011 act. Only with the president's signing of the bill did the FDA, for example, gain the power to deny all food imports from a company that refused to be inspected by the agency. The burden shift means the FDA can now demand that a foreign government accredit all foods the FDA considers high risk, whether sprouts or spices or shrimp. Food companies that pass an FDA verification program will earn the equivalent of the "easy pass" line for trusted passengers at U.S. airports, with their imports getting a presumptive okay and faster processing at FDA ports.[24]

Food safety experts believe that in some large, increasingly sophisticated international governments, and in multinational food companies with worldwide consumer reputations to maintain, these kinds of changes could accomplish great things. Governments such as India and China, which rely on exports as a foreign currency lifeline, are likely to make their systems more transparent and lean on their corporations to comply, said the University of Maryland's Buchanan. China's melamine scandal didn't just bring admonitions from the FDA and USDA, it prompted intense scrutiny from the European Union, the World Health Organization, and others. "They are scrambling to regain the confidence of the food industry," Buchanan said.

And yet. In the years it will take for governments and multinationals to force safer food production, many tainted cargo loads will arrive at U.S. shores. The conflicting principles of commerce and oversight, cat and mouse, of finding concrete revenue to pay for budgetary dreams—those are the realities that lead food safety experts to keep a wary eye on Chilean table grapes, or Thai-farmed shrimp, or Chihuahuan green onions.

The same food safety act that promised so many new powers relies on levels of government competence and unchallenged budget requests that are as realistic as an office of Unicorn Inspections. By the sixth year of the 2011 act's existence, the FDA is supposed to conduct 19,200 inspections of foreign food producers. How many did it actually inspect in foreign countries the year before the act took effect? That would be 354.[25]

There are more than 250,000 foreign entities along the chain linking overseas food to the United States. In the 2013 budget, the FDA asked for a total of ninety-four new full-time employees to work on the foreign food inspections.[26] Even that minimal number has met with fierce resistance. Half of Congress hates the idea of forcing new fees on industry to fund tighter regulation of that same industry. FDA budget requests are prayers that are rarely answered. While the agency pleads for the new money it needs to carry out what Congress ordered it to do, the enormous federal deficit turns the debate each year away from how much to increase and toward the question of how much to cut. Of the FDA's "boots on the ground" tough talk, one seasoned food safety researcher concluded, "It sounds good, when you say it fast."

By July 2013, far enough from election cycles for Obama budget officials to release the detailed new food safety rules, the FDA finally announced two more of the crucial proposals meant to flesh out the modernization act signed in 2011. They gave more precise instructions to food importers about developing plans to prevent pathogens and the recordkeeping required if FDA inspectors came around asking to see the

plans. The rules also launched a certification process for third-party auditors in foreign countries. The new rules would make significant strides
and "build safety into the supply chain" rather than just hoping to "catch
it at the border," said FDA commissioner Dr. Margaret Hamburg.[27] Reporters, though, pressed the FDA officials on what new resources they
would have to enforce the rules. They offered the bureaucratic equivalent
of crossed fingers. President Obama's latest budget had requested some
of the new money required; the rest would have to come from the fees on
American food-handling facilities that Obama proposed and Republicans
still resisted. "Those discussions are ongoing, and I hope will bear fruit,"
Hamburg concluded.[28]

Though federal agents can't possibly eyeball every shipment of food
into the United States, they do take a hard look at a few items. From
among more than ten million food shipments into 320 ports in a recent
year, the FDA rejected just under sixteen thousand items.[29] Some per-
ishables are destroyed on site. But not all of them. Many are simply put
back on the ship. The more audacious importers may try to relabel or
otherwise disguise the items and try again at another U.S. port, while others will seek better odds at a port of a different nation farther down the
food safety chain. "If the U.S. rejects a shipment, it's going to go to some
other country," said Buchanan. "Sooner or later, they'll find a place to
dump it." The high-tech screening systems envisioned by the Food Safety
Modernization Act could in theory collect and connect all the information
about the shipper of that rejected food, marking them down as a bad actor
that needs to be scrutinized with every future cargo. Yet many times U.S.
agents have tried to track down the foreign entities actually responsible
for producing a lot of suspect food only to pursue phantom corporate
names, a warehouse gone out of business in the time it took a container
ship to cross the ocean, or ingredient suppliers deep in the heart of a
nation hostile to outside investigators. Imagine boxes of snack bars with
milk protein boosted by poisonous melamine. Who imported the snacks?
Which company baked them, thousands of miles away? Who supplied the
powdered milk to that bakery? Which dairy farmer trucked in the milk
reduced for that particular batch of powder? What fly-by-night chemical
broker sold that small-time dairy farmer a few bags of cheap additive?
It's enough to make the experts wish for the challenge of a needle in a
haystack, since finding one would be easier.

Consumers of beef and chicken in America have plenty to worry about
in the average food safety year. *E. coli* in undercooked hamburgers, *Salmonella* in chicken left just a little too juicy, *Listeria* lurking in the cold cases

of processed deli meats. But carnivores have far more protection when it comes to imported meat sources than consumers of all the foods overseen by the FDA. Through a combination of successful industry lobbying and the geographic realities of centralized mass animal slaughter, the USDA wields relatively explicit powers when it comes to getting its inspectors' boots inside the doors of overseas meat and poultry producers.

If a Canadian packer, for example, wants to start shipping steaks and burgers south across the border, it would first have to apply for "equivalency" certification from the USDA.[30] The U.S. agency would study the nation's food safety laws and on-site inspection protocols, and while not demanding "identical" procedures, they would require that the system be designed to produce equally safe results. Then the USDA sends its own auditors abroad for full audits of the plants producing the meats headed for export. There are public comment periods for those who want to object or demand more specifics. Even if the Canadian plant passes those tests, it's subject to periodic audits from U.S. personnel, must conduct the same microbiological sample tests as U.S. plants, and must allow every lot of meat to be inspected and tested again by U.S. border agents.[31] "It certainly works better than the FDA," said Christopher Waldrop of the Consumer Federation of America. A former leader of the USDA's FSIS called the foreign auditing system "one of the crown jewels" of U.S. protections.

A late summer *E. coli* scare in Canada in 2012 shows what happens when once-approved companies slip below the high U.S. standards. Montana border inspectors found *E. coli* O157:H7 in samples of beef from an enormous XL Foods plant in Alberta, an operation slaughtering thousands of head of cattle a day and exporting to twenty countries.[32] The recall grew to millions of pounds of Canadian beef, part of the three-billion-plus pounds of foreign meat allowed into the United States each year. As questions multiplied about how long Canadian authorities delayed warning their own consumers of the suspect beef, the plant was "delisted" from the U.S. approval list. That one plant in Alberta handled a third of all of Canada's cattle, and the temporary closure caused a livestock jam to ripple across the provinces.

The power to get those boots on the ground for foreign inspections in beef and chicken plants is only important, of course, if the U.S. government actually uses it. The latest Canadian beef troubles prompted reporters at the dogged *Food Safety News* to ask when was the last time U.S. auditors had been in the Alberta buildings to look around. It turned out they were getting set to go again, on a regularly scheduled trip, when the XL beef started turning up bad at the border.[33] The trouble was, the last such inspection had been back in 2009, three years before. As the reporters kept asking for audit records the USDA somehow left off its websites, they learned the inspection agency had quietly dropped back from annual visits in nearly every country to much longer gaps between trips. Of about thirty-four foreign nations approved to export beef or poultry to the United States, the FSIS was inspecting an average of twenty-six nations each year through 2008. But then the numbers plummeted. For the next three years, the FSIS did in-person checks of just under ten nations a year. In 2011, it got to only three.

How U.S. officials could pull back so radically and still claim to be improving food safety is a mystery solved only by understanding that government agencies hope they can substitute affordable computer modeling for expensive people. Both the USDA and the FDA are shifting important, human-reliant food safety systems to more targeted, risk-based approaches. These shifts combine enormous databases and predictive modeling to make up for the growing gap between the amount of food flooding into U.S. ports and the portions inspectors have time to see for themselves.

The new system is called PREDICT, as a predictably incomprehensible government acronym[34]—Predictive Risk-Based Evaluation for Dynamic Import Compliance Targeting. And that's just the hardware. The software was dubbed MARCS, for "Mission Accomplishment and Regulatory Compliance Services," but since that didn't really mean anything, they tacked on "Imports Entry Review." So in full, that would be MARCS-IER, perhaps to imply that it's definitely more MARCS than the last system.

PREDICT chews up information on a food shipment's invoice, sprinkles in data about the import company and other FDA records, and creates a score for that bundle of goods. Maybe there's been a recent recall of Mexican strawberries, so any other shipments of strawberries from south of the border get a higher—worse—score. Maybe the import company has a good past record with FDA and was granted "equivalency" or something close to it—lower score. The score for that item is compared to hundreds of thousands of other scores generated in the previous thirty days, and the highest-percentile scores get red-flagged for closer human inspection. Food coming in with a low-risk score is largely assumed to be ready for sale and passed through without further frisking.[35]

The FDA's official line is that PREDICT works as promised, with more human inspections resulting in violations because the computers point employees toward the riskiest foods. Yet in describing the system, they also acknowledged they hadn't found time or money to put all their past records on companies into the database; in other words, they were data mining only on the surface. The congressional "fiscal cliff" of early 2013, just one in an ongoing series of surreal deadlines for a very real budget crisis, made pessimists out of those wondering when the FDA could catch up on its own paperwork and make its database current.

As the FDA waits to see when it will get the money to carry out its grand plans and how many years in a row Congress will support the commitment, new contamination worries are creeping into the food safety conversation. Consumer watchdogs are seeing more and more cases of illness and recall from exotic spices and condiments, as an American cooking culture addicted to the Food Network seeks authentic flavors. A hepatitis A scare in the summer of 2013 sickened more than 150 people across the United States after most reported eating a frozen berry mixture sold at discount stores and used to make fruit smoothies and other health-promoting dishes.[36] The berries came from multiple states and countries, making traceback a challenge. Then, a new level of complication: the hepatitis A strain found in samples from many victims matched strains of the virus found only in the Middle East and North Africa. That led to the pomegranate seeds thrown into the berry mix, supplied through Turkey. One simple bag of berries for a smoothie blended the food safety challenges of at least four nations.

The promise and limitations of relying on computer technology to watchdog imported foods were prominently on display in another recent *Salmonella* outbreak that sickened hundreds and resulted in the recall of more than a million pounds of meat.

The CDC's Pulse network, described earlier, functioned as the perfect, tireless add-on to human intelligence that it was designed to be. Late one summer, as the software made their customary scans of illness patterns coming from state and local health departments across America, PulseNet discovered a cluster of *Salmonella* illnesses with the same genetic fingerprints in the Petri dish.[37] CDC officials coordinate with state health departments to send epidemiologists into the field, wielding the exhaustive questionnaires on three hundred commonly eaten foods that can reveal common patterns among the sick. The first batch of questionnaires in the *Salmonella* cases came back with no clear answers, though. The percentages of the ill who had eaten certain suspect foods were no greater than percentages of healthy people who traditionally report eating the same foods within the past week.

Months after the first Pulse patterns emerged, epidemiologists fanned out again, this time to only sixteen of the *Salmonella* patients, to conduct open-ended interviews beyond the usual lists of foods. They quickly found twelve of the sixteen, or 75 percent, had reported eating some kind of deli salami, much higher than the percentages found over years in a healthy population of eaters. A large number said they bought the salami at national warehouse chains, such as Costco, Sam's Club, and others selling in bulk.[38] The epidemiologists jumped on the results and took advantage of more computer technology: the reams of information stored with the membership card numbers of the members-only warehouse chains. With that data, they could isolate precisely the brands of meat purchased, and then work backward through the companies' supplier chain to the distributors and meat processors.

The focus on meat products shifted the burden of investigation to the USDA's FSIS. Investigators descended on plants in Rhode Island and elsewhere. But their microbe tests came up negative. The salami when it first came off the production line was clean. The steps the meat processors used on the meat parts achieved desired "lethality," killing off any remaining germs through fermentation and drying. So the *Salmonella* cases in more than forty states were still a mystery. But the *Salmonella* was clearly in the meats when they left the plant, thus a sweeping recall began. In January 2010, first 1.3 million pounds of salami, and later hundreds of thousands of pounds more, were called back from warehouses and stores around the nation.

Scientists turned to scrutinizing what happened to the salami after the curing rooms and before boxes of products left the shipping dock. When they tested bins of red and black pepper used to crust the salami with a tangy bite, they found the culprit. High percentages of the spice lots were crawling with *Salmonella*. Once the salami was rolled in the pepper, there was no additional "lethality" step to kill remaining pathogens on the product before it went into a package.

Spice companies that supplied the meatpacker called back more than fifty thousand pounds of red pepper in February, and more than fifty thousand pounds of black pepper in March. The peppers were imported from three Asian countries.

From the time the first related cases of *Salmonella* were reported in August 2009 to the time the black pepper was recalled, seven months had passed. Imagine how many different foods across the United States were made with those same suspect sources of pepper, and how much food was consumed in that time.

Spices are one of the newest nightmares for those whose job it is to worry about imported foods. Call it the "We Three Kings" problem. Exotic flavorings of an uncertain provenance, brought as culinary gifts to an eager world of chefs and chef wannabes, then sprinkled in minute amounts across a cornucopia of foods. Figuring out where those Three Kings came from, and what exactly they brought with them, takes the imported food challenge to an infinitely complex level.

There are lethality steps for spices, long known to producers and thoroughly tested. Irradiation, which we'll discuss at more length in a later chapter on the future science of food safety, has been proven to kill microbes in spices without altering flavors or leaving behind radioactivity. Steam treatment of spices also can eliminate many pathogens, though it is trickier to do so without altering the consistency or flavors.

About eight countries supply 75 percent of spices to the United States, and India is the top supplier, said Georgia's Doyle. "If you see how these spices are grown and harvested and transported, you realize there's lots of potential for pathogen contamination,"[39] he said, and studies show a consistently high percentage of spices tainted by *Salmonella*. Other researchers put it another way: imagine the tiny, underdeveloped nations that are home to the most popular spices. Think of local trade workers harvesting, peeling, grinding, sorting, and washing these ancient flavors. And then realize they often are places where tourists don't want to drink the water.

5

DIRTY DISHES: WHAT HAPPENS
TO THE PERPETRATORS?

Jeff Almer's mother was petite but tough. She had beaten lung cancer and survived a brain tumor. Jeff and his four siblings hoped Shirley Almer would live as long as their grandmother, who clung on until 101 years old. Instead, Shirley died at age seventy-two, one day before her doctors intended to release her from a rehabilitation center in time for Christmas at home.[1]

It was peanut butter that killed her.

An investigation taken all the way to the U.S. Capitol would reveal more than blind ignorance was responsible for the shipping of tainted peanuts all over the country in 2008. The chief executives of PCA had been told—dozens of times—that their peanuts were contaminated with *Salmonella*, a potentially deadly pathogen. But instead of cleaning up their plant, they orchestrated an elaborate scheme to ship contaminated peanuts with falsified certificates claiming the nuts were clean and ready for consumption, according to a federal indictment.[2] Time and again, bacteria-laced peanuts—roasted in a plant dotted with rat droppings—were shipped to manufacturers, who used them to make peanut butter crackers, cookies, and snack bars, investigators found.

Nine people, including Shirley Almer, would die.

For four years afterward, the families of the dead waited in anguish. It seemed there would be no consequence. No indictment. No charges. No jail time. The case was lambasted as the prime example of a toothless system in which companies that kill people with tainted products are not punished. This time, total disregard for the safety of the human food supply was exposed by Congress. "Smoking gun" memos were revealed, yet swift punishment did not follow.

Then in February 2013, federal prosecutors released a scathing, seventy-six-count indictment that changed the landscape of foodborne illness investigations. The president of the PCA and three other executives were accused of fooling their customers into believing their peanuts were safe to eat when they allegedly knew otherwise. On top of that, the company was ordering batches of Mexican peanut paste and mixing it into its own product, all the while deceiving its customers by telling them the peanuts were made in the United States, according to the indictment.

Until then, even among the most scandalous food poisonings in American history, criminal charges were not just rare; they had been virtually nonexistent. Here is how it almost always goes: company officials—if the recall was widespread and the food poisonings dire—pay for their actions through tarnished reputations and bankruptcy. Or, if the number of injured is only a handful, and the company is able to secure a confidential settlement with its victims, there are no consequences of substance. No public embarrassment. No nudge to significantly improve safety procedures. No signal to consumers to avoid the brand.

Prosecution of the bad actors who sell contaminated food without regard for human safety is yet another part of the American food safety system that needs work. Demanding more pathogen testing at factories doesn't do much good in the long run unless there are consequences for failed tests and for food shipped despite failed tests. Some safety advocates argue that the U.S. government should put more effort into prosecution after outbreaks, not only to raise safety concerns among American food producers but also to send the signal to foreign countries that there are consequences for shipping unsafe food. The FDA now has the power to oversee foreign third-party contractors that inspect foreign factories, but the federal government has not gone after the domestic audit companies that gave Wright County Egg, PCA, or Jensen Farms glowing ratings before they shipped contaminated foods.

At the start of the Peanut Corporation scandal, it looked as if prosecution was imminent. Drama was high, making it seem unlikely to the public that it would take years before the wheels of justice started rolling. At a hearing before a congressional committee in 2009, about two months after Shirley Almer and eight others died, U.S. Representative Greg Walden of Oregon held up a clear jar of contaminated cookies and crackers made with peanuts from PCA and asked its executives, "Would either of you be willing to take the lid off and eat any of these products?"[3] For exaggerated dramatic effect, the jar was wrapped in yellow crime scene tape.

PCA chief executive Stewart Parnell responded by pleading the Fifth. "Mr. Chairman and members of the committee, on advice of my counsel, I respectfully decline to answer your questions based on the protections afforded me under the U.S. Constitution," he said.

Parnell was clearly rattled. Witnesses recalled his hands shaking. After repeating the statement several times, Parnell—in Washington under congressional subpoena—was allowed to leave.

Congressional investigators had uncovered incriminating emails showing Parnell apparently knew the peanuts were contaminated and, concerned about profits, still ordered the plant to "turn them loose." The emails and other documents were revealed at the U.S. House Energy and Commerce Committee hearing, crowded with relatives of those who died after eating contaminated peanut butter products. Among those in the audience were some who had been sickened, including a three-year-old boy who grew ill eating peanut butter crackers.

In one email, Blakely, Georgia, plant manager Sammy Lightsey responded with "uh-oh" after being told an outside lab had found *Salmonella* bacteria on the products. In another email, Parnell wrote to Lightsey that the positive *Salmonella* tests were "costing us huge $$$$$ and causing obviously a huge lapse in time from the time we pick up peanuts until the time we can invoice." And later, even after federal officials determined PCA was the source of the outbreak sickening hundreds of people, Parnell sent an email to FDA officials begging them to let the company keep operating. We "desperately at least need to turn the raw peanuts on our floor into money," he wrote.[4]

Other documents and congressional testimony showed the peanut company fired the private lab it had been using to test products because the lab was returning too many positive *Salmonella* tests. An official at J. Leek Associates laboratory, Michelle Pronto, testified at the hearing that when she informed the Georgia plant manager about one of the positive tests, he told her the product was already on "a truck headed to Utah."

The scheme that kept the company running and ended up sickening people across the country was much worse than even was revealed on Capitol Hill, according to the federal government's indictment.

Parnell and his associates shipped roasted peanut products to numerous other manufacturers before they were tested for *Salmonella*, investigators found. Worse, when it was discovered the peanuts were contaminated, they did not tell their customers. They accomplished this by sending altered "certificates of analysis" along with the shipments that included test results from previous lots of peanuts. The company would take several samples for testing from the same lot of peanut paste, so if the product cleared testing, they would have a handful of "clean" certificates. Then they assigned those certificates to lots of product that hadn't even been made yet, investigators claim. Parnell's attorney has said Parnell never intentionally harmed anyone.

PCA sent two to three tanker truckloads of peanut paste per week to a North Carolina customer that made peanut butter crackers. Part of the alleged "conspiracy" included product testing procedures that PCA executives knew would result in two things: most of the paste shipped to that cracker plant was never tested at all, and every shipment was sent with a "false and misleading" certificate of analysis, according to the federal indictment.

This couldn't have been the "state-of-the-art food safety techniques" the company was bragging about in a brochure, calling itself "The Processor of the World's Finest Peanut Products."

The same North Carolina plant making peanut butter crackers also was duped into thinking all of its peanut paste was made with American-grown peanuts. In fact, PCA was buying Mexican peanut paste by the truckload and mixing it into the customer's order—oftentimes at a ratio of up to 50 percent, according to the federal indictment.

The emails between company executives uncovered by the federal investigation were damning. In one, Michael Parnell told his brother Stewart that the company could provide fictitious testing analysis to customers if needed. "Truthfully if a customer called and needed one that was for say two pallets or so they would create one. Most of the time smaller people will accept one produced with your company heading on it that looked professionally done. The girl in TX was very good at white-out," he wrote.

In another, Stewart Parnell wrote, "Shit, just ship it," after he was told *Salmonella* test results were not ready yet and would cause a delay for the customer.

And another: An employee advised before shipping an order of peanut meal, "They need to air hose the top off though because they are covered in dust and rat crap." It wasn't the only mention of rodents in company emails.

Mary Wilkerson, who began as PCA's office receptionist and eventually became quality assurance manager, answered "MICE!" to a coworker who emailed asking, "Where do you think all this [*sic*] coliform positives are coming from? Would you say it is the negative air pressure in the plant bringing in airborne pathogens? Like over that rancid peanut butter along the fence?"

In a 2008 email exchange regarding questions from the FDA about why a customer had rejected its shipment of peanuts, Stewart Parnell and fellow executive Daniel Kilgore apparently agreed to give false information. They decided to tell FDA investigators the shipment was rejected because the peanuts were not cut to the right size. The truth was that the nuts possibly contained metal fragments. "We all need to have our stories straight if and when we are questioned by the FDA," Kilgore wrote.

Kilgore was the first executive named in the indictment to cooperate with federal authorities. He pleaded guilty to conspiracy to commit fraud, conspiracy to introduce adulterated and misbranded food into interstate commerce, introducing adulterated food into interstate commerce with the intent to defraud, plus several other charges. His attorney declined to comment.

After the indictment was released, Michael Moore, U.S. attorney for the Middle District of Georgia, said the defendants "cared less about the quality of the food they were providing to the American people and more about the quantity of money they were gathering while disregarding food safety."[5]

In one email from 2008, Parnell berated employees for wasting 1,374 pounds of peanut products left over from production. "I am not sure anyone down there quite understands how SERIOUS this is. . . . These are not peanuts you are throwing away every day. It is money. It is money. It is money. It is God Damn Money."

The law firm representing Stewart Parnell had this to say after the indictment: "As this matter progresses it will become clear that Mr. Parnell never intentionally shipped or intentionally caused to be shipped any tainted food products capable of harming PCA's customers."[6] It may be years longer before consumers and regulators get any satisfactory answers about what really happened—and who knew it—inside the peanut plants.

When it comes to testing food products before shipping, proper protocol is to throw out any batch that tests positive and figure out the problem. When a sample from a batch tests positive, that doesn't mean the entire batch is contaminated. Multiple tests from the same batch could come up with varied results.

The testing process is particularly tricky with foods such as peanuts. *Salmonella* bacteria doesn't spread evenly; tests aren't going to find it on every peanut. It depends on the sample, so it's possible, even probable, that a sample from one batch of peanuts could come out clean while another sample from the same batch could turn up contaminated with *Salmonella*. If PCA received a positive test, the company at times had the same batch of peanuts tested by another lab or the same lab in the hope the second test would find a clean spot in the pile and come back negative for *Salmonella*, according to the indictment.

The FDA's Office of Criminal Investigation began the probe into the Georgia peanut plant, which led to the FBI executing search warrants. FDA inspectors visited PCA's plant in January 2009 and found at least a dozen samples from the company's production were contaminated in 2007 and 2008, but the corporation did not clean up the problem. The company filed for bankruptcy in 2009.[7] After four years, a federal grand jury finally convened in Georgia in the fall of 2012 to hear testimony about the outbreak.

Many of the products shipped from the plant in Blakely, Georgia, ended up as jumbo-sized buckets of peanut butter used in school cafeterias, nursing homes, and rehabilitation centers. The list of potentially contaminated products in 2008 was in the thousands, the recalls extensive and costly. The list of recalled products went on for pages. Among those jumbo-sized tubs of peanut butter laced with *Salmonella* bacteria was one purchased by a rehabilitation center in Minnesota.

After treatments that eliminated her brain tumor, Shirley Almer's doctors sent her to a rehab center next to the University of Minnesota Hospital that was supposed to help her get stronger. She wasn't up to her usual strength, and she was extra picky about what she would eat, refusing almost any nourishment but for chicken and peanut butter toast. The rehabilitation center kept an industrial-sized tub of peanut butter for its residents, and Shirley's daughter Ginger toasted a slice of bread and smeared it with peanut butter for her mother almost every day. And each day, Shirley would nibble a few bites. Only a few bites.

At first, Shirley was outperforming doctors' expectations as she recovered from radiation to treat the tumor and the damage left behind by seizures brought on by the mass in her brain. Physicians said she might not regain the use of her arms and legs. But she did. After about two months in the rehab center, she was released to her family. She spent weekdays with Ginger in Brainerd, Minnesota, and then on weekends she would go to her own home in Perham, about an hour away. Her five children took turns watching her on weekends.

Just before Thanksgiving, it was Jeff's turn to watch his mother. She had been getting weaker and was doing worse than when she left the rehab center. She wasn't eating much, was losing weight, and was sleeping more than she should. She was too weak to walk.

"I literally carried her out of her house for the last time," Jeff recalled. At Brainerd Hospital, she was diagnosed with severe dehydration and a urinary tract infection; there was an infection in her blood, but it was unclear what exactly was wrong with her. No one mentioned *Salmonella* yet. No one in her family had any clue it was food poisoning that was killing her. Doctors tried to clear the infections and said she could go home December 22 to spend Christmas with her family.

Jeff was shoveling snow when his sister called December 21, 2008. The ice storm was fierce. "You better get up here," Ginger said. "They don't expect her to last the day."

When Jeff and his wife arrived at the hospital in Brainerd, nurses were wheeling out a cart of refreshments: finger sandwiches and cookies. He knew it was what they must give people who are hanging around waiting for someone to die. "It will be OK. You can let go," he said to his mom through tears. "She was hanging on just for us," Jeff said. "She had fought and fought and fought. I hugged and kissed her. It felt like a dramatic movie scene, and I was living it."

Shirley was having trouble breathing because of fluid in her lungs. The doctors were correct—she didn't last the day.

Her family thought she had died of pneumonia. On Christmas Day, four days later, Jeff opened the shirt and GPS unit his mother had bought for him before she took a turn for the worse. The emptiness he felt consumed him.

After the holidays, on a day in January about three weeks after Shirley died, the Minnesota health department called Ginger and asked if she had a few minutes to talk about what Shirley had eaten in the months before she died. The hospital had reported to the state health department that Shirley had *Salmonella*, although her family hadn't been told. Ginger mentioned her mother ate mostly chicken and peanut butter at the end of her life.

Several days later, Jeff noticed an Associated Press blurb in the *Minneapolis Star Tribune* about a *Salmonella* outbreak that so far was linked to the death of a northern Minnesota woman. He called his sister, and she called the state health department. Yes, health authorities told her, that's your mother you read about, and we're sorry you had to find out like this. "If it's any consolation, what you told us she ate has been key to solving this outbreak," Jeff recalled a health official saying.

About a month later, in February 2009, Jeff testified at the congressional hearings into the peanut butter bacteria outbreak that killed Shirley and eight others. He assumed, until that day, that the plant that shipped the contaminated peanuts was simply careless. But when congressional staff released the smoking-gun emails, showing PCA chief executive Parnell apparently ordered the peanuts shipped even though he was told they were tainted, Jeff was outraged. "I was completely dumbfounded and shocked," he said.

Jeff turned to the son of another victim. "Can you believe this shit?" he asked him. "This guy is going to be in prison in about a month." And he thought to himself, "What would happen to me if I just got up right now and went over and gave that guy one straight shot to the chops?" He remembered Parnell's hands were shaking. Outside the hearing room, Jeff told a television reporter he had a message for Parnell. "I hope you never get Alzheimer's because I want you to remember this day for the rest of your life," he said.

By the time the grand jury convened in Georgia, Jeff had met with investigators from the FBI and the U.S. Department of Justice more than once. "To me, it's nine murders," Jeff said he told them.

Shirley's children joined other families in a lawsuit against Peanut Corporation, which filed for bankruptcy. The families of the nine victims were each awarded a piece of $12 million available, divided, to put it bluntly, on the calculated value of each of their lives. Shirley's life, negotiators determined, was worth $98,000.

"They hadn't seen what my mom did in beating cancer," Jeff said. "This was a woman planning to go home for Christmas. That was stolen from her."

The 2008 to 2009 *Salmonella* peanut butter outbreak sickened more than seven hundred people and spread to forty-six states.[8] Nearly four thousand products linked to the tainted peanuts were recalled. President Barack Obama promised a top-to-bottom look at America's food safety system. He was particularly concerned about children, mentioning his daughter Sasha ate peanut butter "probably three times a week."

As with many of its more sensitive issues, the FDA responds reluctantly and obscurely to questions about its criminal investigation process. And it responds in writing. The FDA declines to describe how it decides who is worthy of pursuit, or how often it tries to make a case.

If a criminal investigation of Peanut Corporation executives was slow and difficult, any case against product manufacturers that used peanut ingredients from the company was a stretch, especially since those companies allegedly were getting falsified certificates of analysis with their deliveries. Dozens of companies had received shipments of peanuts to use in ice cream, crackers, bars, and other snacks, and many of those companies were sued along with PCA.

Attorney Justin Prochnow, among the nation's most well-known food and diet supplement safety lawyers, represented an energy bar manufacturer that used nuts from PCA. When lawsuits start flying, the food chain generally goes as it did in this case: the energy bar company sought reimbursement from the manufacturer that made the faulty ingredient, and that manufacturer sought reimbursement from PCA. It's often the case that four or five food manufacturers are involved in the finishing of one product that, like an energy bar, might have ten to fifteen ingredients. In most cases, there is no evidence manufacturers meant to make anyone sick, or that they completely disregarded safety standards while knowing people would get sick. "Intentional fraud is the only time where you are going to see the FDA take criminal action," Prochnow said.[9]

Just as felony charges are rare, so are misdemeanors. Many food safety advocates wish the government would pursue lesser charges rather than none at all. Even if food company owners who sickened people faced no jail time for their actions, misdemeanor charges would send a message—and the public would hear about it. But in general, federal prosecutors seek evidence of willful negligence to elevate cases to felonies, which makes them worth pursuing.

Two years after the cantaloupe outbreak that killed thirty-three people in 2011, federal prosecutors announced misdemeanor charges against two longtime family farmers from rural Colorado. Legal experts had doubted the charges would ever come, unless food safety officials intended to make a political statement that so many deaths could not go unpunished.

The decision not to prosecute the outbreak as a felony, experts said, stemmed from the fact there was no evidence that brothers Eric and Ryan Jensen meant to harm anyone, or knew they had a problem. They had hired a third-party auditor to inspect their farm and had received a glowing report. Fatal flaws in harvest—mainly using a dirty potato sorter and holding melons in water baths—might be considered negligent, but perhaps not willfully negligent. Agricultural experts who talked to the Jensen family said the brothers actually believed changes in harvest procedure in 2011 would make melons safer.[10]

No evidence has emerged during lawsuit fact-finding or congressional queries that the Jensens knew of any dangers from their cantaloupes before state and federal investigators tracked *Listeria* to their farm. The Jensens bought a used potato-sorting machine not designed for cantaloupe use, which allowed water to pool dangerously and helped spread the *Listeria*, the FDA said. The third-party auditor noted the Jensens stopped using antibacterial agents in a new one-pass, clean-water washing system since criticized by others, but the auditor did not suggest they change it.

Ryan Jensen and others at the farm told University of California–Davis cantaloupe expert Trevor Suslow that they believed their new system was an improvement over past packing methods. Though Suslow disagreed, he acknowledged there was no definitive statement in FDA growing guidelines on a single safe method of cleaning, cooling, or packing.

Such ambiguity from the FDA makes prosecution difficult, if not impossible. Food and drug regulations provide misdemeanor and felony charges for cases of "adulterated" food, which includes selling contaminated food. The mere presence of an adulterant on food can justify the charges, regardless of intent. Misdemeanors can result in fines and up to a year in jail.

To elevate a prosecution to a felony, federal officials would have needed evidence the Jensens knew what they were doing was dangerous, or knew they had contamination and delivered melons anyway, said Amanda Hitt, an attorney and director of the Food Integrity Campaign in Washington, D.C. "There are elements for a felony where the 'knowing' element has to be there. Is a jury really going to find that?" Hitt asked.

Among the few food-poisoning outbreaks that resulted in a criminal conviction was the case against juicemaker Odwalla, which sold apple juice tainted with *E. coli* in 1996. Odwalla—the company but not individual executives—pleaded guilty to federal criminal charges in 1998 after the juice killed a Denver toddler and sickened more than sixty others. The California juicemaker was sentenced to five years' probation and was forced to pay a $1.5 million fine after pleading guilty to sixteen misdemeanor charges for "delivering adulterated food products."[11]

A grand jury inquiry into the food poisoning found Odwalla had contracts with suppliers to use only apples picked from trees, not fallen fruit that could be contaminated by animal feces. But the company didn't verify what suppliers provided. Odwalla did not pasteurize its juice by heating it to bacteria-killing temperatures before the outbreak. Now it does. Earlier in 1996, the U.S. Army rejected Odwalla juice because the company's plant-sanitation program did "not adequately assure product wholesomeness for military consumers."[12]

The largest fine for violating U.S. food-and-drug law didn't result from a food-poisoning case but from a case of fraud—a baby food company advertising sugar water as 100 percent apple juice. In 1987, a grand jury investigation led to a $2 million fine and 215 violations of federal law against Beech-Nut Nutrition Corporation for selling phony apple juice. The juice was apple-flavored water with corn syrup and beet sugar.

Two Beech-Nut executives were sentenced to jail time and community service.[13]

But what about in cases when there is perhaps no fraud or conspiracy, just a lackadaisical disregard for safety?

Another of the United States' most egregious food-illness outbreaks, and one of the most disgusting, has resulted in no criminal charges. Reading inspection reports written after the Wright County Egg farm outbreak of 2010 is enough even to make the most strong-stomached among us feel queasy.

FDA investigators found decaying mice, chicken carcasses, and manure piled so high that the chicken-house door wouldn't shut. A month after that outbreak, owners of the Wright County Egg farm were lambasted by the U.S. House Energy and Commerce Committee. The bad eggs sickened hundreds of people across the country. The farm received 426 positive results for *Salmonella* between 2008 and 2010, yet it continued its practices, according to documents obtained by the House committee.[14] The government's criminal investigation into the outbreak, which involved a grand jury in Iowa, resulted in a bribery conviction of a manager at the egg farm. But no one has been charged directly for causing the outbreak that sickened so many. Former DeCoster Farms manager Tony Wasmund pleaded guilty in 2012 to conspiring to bribe a federal inspector to allow the sale of restricted eggs. Wasmund was accused of authorizing spending $300 in petty cash for use as a bribe for a USDA inspector months before the outbreak.[15]

Wasmund had been informed of Iowa State University lab reports in the months before the outbreak showing *Salmonella* was found in the internal organs of dead chickens at the farm, according to federal documents.

Austin "Jack" DeCoster, who had built an egg dynasty, gave up control of egg operations in Iowa, Maine, and Ohio in 2011. Other companies purchased control of the operations.[16]

Food-illness attorney Fred Pritzker, one of the country's most popular lawyers for victims of foodborne illness, called the government's lack of prosecution in the egg outbreak "mystifying." "This is willful negligence," said Pritzker, of Minneapolis. "It's kind of like being a drunk driver, or a careless driver—I'm not trying to hurt anybody; I'm just a moron."[17]

Drunk drivers are prosecuted. Yet people who produce food for human consumption in the most deplorable of conditions are not. Numerous times, Pritzker said, he has been taking the deposition of a safety executive for a food producer and thought, "Are you kidding me? Are you imbeciles?"

An attorney for the DeCoster family said it was "very false and misleading" to suggest the egg company owners were willfully negligent. Unlike the peanut butter case, the Wright County Egg case has no allegations of a coverup, or falsified lab results, or failing to provide notice to customers that bad product had been shipped, said lawyer Jerry Crawford.

In one recent case, Pritzker was representing a seventeen-year-old girl who lost her kidney function after going out for a steak dinner at a popular chain restaurant with her family to celebrate her good grades. Pritzker couldn't name the chain because the company negotiated a confidentiality agreement when it paid the teenager's family in a private settlement.

The steak she ate was "mechanically tenderized," a process of stabbing the meat with needles to make it feel and taste like a better cut of meat. Many steaks at chain restaurants are mechanically tenderized, experts said. The problem with the process is that beef often has *E. coli* on its surface, and the needles that tenderize it can push the bacteria inside the meat. Normally, it's safe to eat steak that's pink on the inside as long as the outside is seared to kill off any bacteria. The inside of the steak is clean—but not when you push the bacteria from the surface to the inside of the meat.

Mechanically tenderized steak has been the source of numerous *E. coli* outbreaks across the country. In Pritzker's case involving the seventeen-year-old girl, he sued the manufacturer that tenderized the meat. Under questioning during a deposition, Pritzker learned the company knew its spray equipment meant to kill pathogens was not working properly. They had experts look at it, and they were told it wasn't functioning as it should. Still, they continued selling the mechanically tenderized steaks.

Neither the meat producer nor the tenderizer went bankrupt paying settlements to two victims Pritzker represented. Insurance paid the claims, as is usually the case. And as is usually the case, the companies insisted on confidentiality agreements to prevent the lawyers or clients from talking about what happened. The confidentiality protects the company from public scrutiny and keeps food safety advocates in the dark.

It's by no means a guarantee that companies forced to pay because of an outbreak won't do it again. In fact, many of the big meat producers have been involved in numerous outbreaks. The secrecy of the process protects them. And if insurance is paying, the worst that might happen are increased premiums. Imagine a company that makes billions of dollars in annual sales. Paying a few million to people who nearly died eating their steak isn't going to break the company.

But it's not as simple as that, said Pritzker, who has been representing food illness victims and families for twenty years. It's a common belief among food producers that it won't happen to them. "I think a lot of companies hate the idea both morally and financially of harming the public," he said. "But I think there is a huge belief amongst most companies that it won't happen to us, it hasn't happened to us and we have good systems." If companies would invest more up front on safety protocol, they could prevent the outbreaks that end up costing them exponentially more, Pritzker said.

"These companies hate like hell to have an outbreak. It's the worst thing that can happen to their business. Do they have any ongoing consequences? Never as much as they should. There is not a single case that I have been involved in that didn't involve some egregious conduct on the part of some-body in the food distribution chain. Make them pay. Make them have some skin in the game."

Number one on most companies' list of what to do in case of an outbreak is call a public relations firm. Minimizing the damage is the goal. Compa-nies have this on their side when it comes to public exposure: "The public's memory is very weak," Pritzker said.

Experts point to two main reasons that criminal prosecution after food-borne illness outbreaks are rare. First, federal prosecutors have limited resources, so they shy away from cases that might be harder to prove, cases with an unfamiliar pathogen or unusual food source. The second theory is that federal regulators and the industry are too friendly, a relationship that evolved through years of working together. Each time the FDA or USDA creates a regulation, it works with the industry, holding public comment periods throughout a long collaborative effort. Relatively few companies control the meat production in this country, and they work closely with the federal government through their trade association. USDA inspectors are stationed full time in factories. They get to know each other well.

"Relationships get forged and I think that closeness tends to obscure prosecutorial decisions," Pritzker said. "The idea is not to protect the indus-try. The idea is to prevent foodborne illness. Sometimes you need to crush a few egos and a few skulls to create that message."

Criminal proceedings have become so unlikely that no one seemed to expect anything of the sort after Colorado's cantaloupe *Listeria* outbreak, quickly traced to melons grown by the Jensen brothers.

"It would seem unfair to go after the Jensens as an example when you haven't gone after anybody in twenty years," said Bill Marler of Seattle, the nation's most well-known food illness lawyer. Felony charges against the Jensens might have been a stretch, but prosecution on lighter misde-meanor charges would send a message to large food companies to focus on safety, Marler said. Jensen Farms' distributor and auditor, Frontera and PrimusLabs, should have been legally forced to tighten standards after the outbreak, Marler said. "When companies change behavior is when they are held up to public scrutiny," he said. Two years after the Colorado out-break, some families clung to a desire for the farm to see tougher justice, but reports of federal interest were vague and sporadic. Some news outlets predicted charges against the Jensens in 2012, a year after the outbreak, but the calendar year turned without a change.

Along with public scrutiny, lawsuits with the potential to put companies out of business can also inspire change. Lawsuits are the main form of punishment in this country for food producers who make people ill, and the targets of those lawsuits are expanding. The three prime targets of lawsuits in the cantaloupe *Listeria* outbreak had just $17 million in liability coverage for more than 130 illness cases that could easily cost more than $100 million in treatment and lost income. "It's not going to be anywhere near enough to compensate all the victims," said Pritzker, who represented some of the *Listeria* victims.

The lack of available compensation led to threats to make new legal targets out of grocery stores, distributors, and auditing labs. "If they can get the deep pockets in, they're going to get them in," Denver lawyer Prochnow said. Grocery stores have a history of trying to protect themselves from lawsuits. How could they expect to know the safety history of each of the thousands of items on their shelves, they argue?

Colorado-based Natural Grocers by Vitamin Cottage pushed state legislation, which was not successful, to protect grocers from liability in merely passing on products made by others. Colorado outbreak investigators linked seven *Salmonella* cases from PCA in 2009 to peanut butter made onsite at Vitamin Cottage stores, apparently using the tainted peanuts. The bill's sponsors in the state legislature thought they were protecting rural grocers from spurious lawsuits; they say that when they learned that it would be a major change in liability law, they killed the bill.

Vitamin Cottage spokesman Alan Lewis said the initial intent of the legislation was to help small businesses that currently have no protection—not to absolve them of any responsibility. "Any good retailer takes responsibility for what they sell and makes good on any deficiency or problem with the product," he said. "That's different than betting your business on every can of soup that you sell."[18]

Grocery stores and other retailers argue that the trial attorneys who get between them and customers end up costing everyone more money. Supermarket food typically has a 1 percent markup that goes toward the store's insurance bill. If customers who were sold bad food complained directly to the store instead of hiring a lawyer, the store could settle the claim on its own, they argue. The legal battle that ensues after an attorney gets involved might result in more money in the lawyer's pocket, but not much more for the consumer than if the store had handled it directly, grocery store owners said.

And deadly outbreaks are expensive. After a spinach outbreak in 2006, about $100 million was spent to settle 110 lawsuits. Attorneys' fees vary widely but generally are in the range of 15 percent to 30 percent or more of settlements.

State laws vary governing who has liability for bad products. Some states, such as California, allow more companies in a food chain to be targets for claims, with few limits on awards. Colorado law makes it harder to sue stores in addition to the producer where the defect started. Plaintiffs must show a retailer contributed to the flaw in the food.

In the cantaloupe *Listeria* lawsuits, which numbered in the dozens, attorneys considered going after retailers for not demanding tougher farm audits, failing to test for pathogens themselves, and failing to wash the fruit one more time before sale. But grocery store owners say going after them is not entirely fair—it's unreasonable to hold grocery stores responsible for the safety of every item on their shelves.

"They have to rely on manufacturers to take care of that end of business and to make sure food items are ready for customer sale when they get them," said Mary Lou Chapman, president of the Rocky Mountain Food Industry Association, which represents more than three hundred grocery stores in Colorado and Wyoming. Chapman supported the Colorado bill that would have protected grocers unless they caused the contamination, or knew it was there when sold.

Yet some food safety advocates say it's time for grocers to take more responsibility than that, especially with foods that cause repeated damage. Hamburger, unpasteurized dairy, spinach, cantaloupes, and other products have often been at the heart of dangerous outbreaks. "At some point, the grocery store has to make a legal or moral decision: 'We're not responsible for the food we sold these people,'" Marler said.

The weight of responsibility finally grew palpable to everyone involved in the Jensen cantaloupe outbreak on a crisp, early fall day in downtown Denver in 2013, more than two years after harvested melons rolled through *Listeria*-laden water in a dusty farm shed. Eric and Ryan Jensen shuffled into a cavernous federal courtroom, shackled at the wrists, fourth-generation farmers whose alleged crime started with a seed planter. The brothers were advised of six misdemeanor charges each of introducing adulterated food into interstate commerce. Each count carried a possible penalty of up to a year in prison, and up to $250,000 in fines. They pleaded not guilty, but shortly after indicated they had reached a deal with prosecutors to enter a guilty plea. Days later, the Jensens sued their third-party auditor for failing to point out any of the problems investigators eventually found, a legal maneuver that promised an escalation of food safety fingerpointing for years to come.

The Jensens declined to talk to reporters, as they had since a wire service photographer had found a bewildered Eric Jensen kicking at unharvested cantaloupe out in his fields, late in the summer of 2011. The Jensens' attorneys emphasized at the courthouse that the brothers had cooperated with food safety investigators from the beginning, and they felt sorrow for the victims of *Listeria*.

Jeni Exley watched the federal judge discuss bond conditions with the Jensens from her spot on a stiff, wooden bench near the back. Her father, Herb Stevens, and the contents of the family refrigerator had been a key link in the fast state investigation that led officials directly to the Jensens. Herb's listeriosis led to two years in a nursing home, and his eventual death, but he was never listed among the thirty-three "official" deaths because of the long delay.

Exley cried quietly outside the courthouse as the Jensens signed bond papers and hurried to a waiting car. "I wanted to humanize this for me," she said. She had never seen the brothers, even in photographs. "I'm glad they were charged. I don't think they did anything on purpose, but I think they had very sloppy farming practices."

The U.S. District Attorney's charges against the Jensens quoted numerous FDA documents and experts in building the case. Five days later, the months-long feud among national leaders culminated in the first shutdown of the federal government in seventeen years. The FDA furloughed 45 percent of its staff, nearly all in food oversight, according to Food Safety News. The agency acknowledged its routine inspections of food operations in the United States would drop to zero—hundreds canceled every week—as long as the shutdown lasted. The CDC, meanwhile, had to send home nine thousand of its thirteen thousand employees. It soon brought back just a dozen—to help seek the source of a widespread outbreak of *Salmonella* in raw chicken.

II

HOW TO FEED YOUR FAMILY SAFELY AND SANELY

6

HANDLE WITH CARE
(AND BLEACH)[1]

Let's call it "defensive eating." The government, food producers, and food packagers all have their vital roles in delivering safer food to Americans, and other chapters in this book hold them to account. But food safety experts say consumers also have a responsibility in making sure the food they buy and serve is safe to eat. It's like this: homeowners aren't to blame if a burglar steals their jewelry, but police still warn people to lock their doors.

The following pages can help you lock pathogens out of your kitchen.

Some of the advice comes from the world of science. Safety experts, splashing and cooking and swabbing for bacteria in university test kitchens, are reconsidering some of the basic tenets of produce handling. The worst foodborne illness outbreak in modern times had the effect of scaring farmers, government inspectors, and home economists into faster action. Before the cantaloupe *Listeria* outbreak in 2011, many people thought nothing of grabbing a melon from the fridge and slicing right into it. Consumer advocates didn't make a big deal about washing melons. Now, most people would at least rinse it before slicing, and food scientists say some people—particularly the very young, old, pregnant, or immune compromised—should wash a melon's porous, pocked rind with soapy water, then pat it dry.

Food safety advice is changing as the world grapples with illness outbreaks, not just from undercooked meat but from spinach, sprouts, tomatoes, and peppers. "It's scary for those of us who give advice, because our world's been rocked," said Lydia Medeiros, a consumer food safety researcher at Ohio State University. "We want to give people good, honest, clear advice. And sometimes we don't know."

Colorado State University was among the laboratories quickly taking the lead in researching safer growing and handling techniques for cantaloupes in 2011. The challenges range from the high tech to the mundane and show just how befuddled even the experts can get by a sudden new development. One of the early ideas discussed by CSU experts, in collaboration with colleagues in the cantaloupe industry, was a new sticker for every cantaloupe telling consumers to thoroughly scrub the netted rind, according to Marisa Bunning, assistant professor for extension and food safety at CSU. But stickers don't stick to cantaloupes, for the same reasons the bumpy rind is a cozy home for pathogens such as *Listeria*.

"What I've learned is that cantaloupes are a challenge, and we've got to readdress it," Bunning said. "We don't know what the best practices would have been to tell consumers to avoid becoming sick. That's why we'll set up experiments."

At an Ohio State University lab, researchers watched pathogens enter tiny pores on spinach leaves and then contaminate a dangerously large area of food. Then they wondered what that meant for an apple or pear that has rolled off the counter and bounced on the floor. The mushy, bruised part of the fruit is more likely to harbor bacteria, so it's best to cut off not just the bruised section but also the area around it just to make sure.

For cantaloupes and other produce with a rind or peel, researchers need to know more about whether pathogens use surface pores or scars to contaminate the fruit or are spread to the inside when a knife is drawn through the whole fruit. The research is tempered by the realities of life in American kitchens. It's highly unlikely an eighty-five-year-old woman is going to hold a four-pound cantaloupe under running water for the long minutes it takes to scrub the whole surface.

Although food safety experts are suggesting more vigilance and consumer responsibility, they warn against becoming obsessed. "We know that there is an inherent risk in all the foods that we consume," said Therese Pilonetti, who manages the Colorado health department's grocery-store-inspection unit. Use common sense, she urges. Even in Pilonetti's line of work, where she hears the worst of what can go on in the farm-to-table food chain, she doesn't bother bagging every item of produce when grocery shopping—she doesn't want to waste so much plastic. She does make sure meat goes in a separate grocery bag from produce, and she washes down her kitchen with a bleach-water solution. She uses tap water and a scrub brush to clean fruits and vegetables.

Safety advocates, including Jean Halloran, director of food policy initiatives for the advocacy arm of *Consumer Reports*, are eager for the U.S. FDA to release new growing guidelines for problem produce— cantaloupe, leafy greens, and tomatoes, for starters—as required by the Food Safety Modernization Act. "In our view, the food that comes to the consumer should be safe to eat, especially stuff that you will eat raw," Halloran says. "But the consumer needs to realize we don't live in a perfect world."

Pregnant women, families with young children, the elderly, and those with compromised immunity should take extra precaution, according to Halloran, but the rest of the public shouldn't worry too much. "Generally, these bugs are not wildly long-lived and hardy. You don't have to become crazy for this. Some people don't pay any attention at all, and that's when you can have a problem."

Ever wondered if you need to scrub the banana peel before you eat the banana? Or if rinsing chicken before you cook it washes off bacteria or just splashes it around your kitchen? Do you really need to wash "prewashed" spinach? How long can the leftovers stay out on the counter while you watch the Packers and the Patriots go into overtime? The answers are not as obvious as your mother's wisdom once told you. Nor are they set in stone. One serious food-illness outbreak can upend years of assumptions in a university lab. But in this chapter, we've called upon national experts to walk us from the grocery aisles, through the kitchen, and all the way to the compost heap.

WHAT TO LOOK FOR AT THE GROCERY STORE

How many times have you grabbed the milk first, wandered over to the bakery aisle, checked the price on the latest Adam Sandler DVD, asked a few questions at the seafood counter, searched high and low for canned artichokes, and then realized your milk isn't cold anymore?

A little terrain mapping of your regular grocery store is a good way to head off some food-illness dangers before you've even paid for the food. Grocery chains hire PhDs in human behavior and marketing to make your visit as labyrinthine and long as possible. More time in the store means more dollars in the till. Fight back with a little basic understanding about where they put the popular stuff, where they put the fresh stuff, and where they put the dangerous stuff.

Shop for dry goods first. You can take all day and even fit in that movie. Pasta, breads, canned items, the massive cereal aisle, all the bathroom needs like tissue and shampoo and toothpaste. With the cans, you probably remember a parent's warning not to buy any cans that bulge outward, an unnatural result that can be an indicator of contaminants growing inside. But also keep an eye out for dents—they may be the result of an innocent drop or ding, but the dents can create a weak spot for outside bacteria to penetrate the can.

When that part of the list is done, cruise through the cooler aisles stacked with milk, cheese, eggs, and fresh meat. And now that you're standing near the chicken parts, look up and realize why they hang rollers of clear plastic bags that seem to belong more in the produce aisles. Many home economists recommend bagging your fresh meat for an extra barrier between the meat packages and anything in your cart that might be consumed raw. If you're planning to use the same hand to pick out fresh produce, slide your hand inside the empty bag first, grab the meat package with the bag as a glove, and invert the bag as you put it in your cart. Just because you're paranoid doesn't mean all those food pathogens aren't really out to get you. Easy steps like these can keep you mindful of food safety without pushing your behavior into the nut aisle.

Some consumer advisers will nudge meat lovers toward a grocery store's fresh butcher counter if they insist on continuing to eat ground beef. They might recommend asking the store's butcher to take an intact cut of beef, such as top sirloin or a chuck roast, and grind it on site into hamburger. It's true this avoids the likelihood of buying hamburger made from grinded beef "trim" gathered from cows raised in a half-dozen states and foreign countries, a process that multiplies the hazards of *E. coli* by mashing all the "outside" beef surfaces into a ground core where pathogens are harder to cook out safely. At least one specialty grocer warns, however, that those butcher counters aren't always hazard free, either. They are only as good as the sanitary habits of the butcher and any assistants, handling multiple cuts of beef under pressure of consumer time and demands. Reconsider frozen meat. One small chain sells ground bison burgers, from buffalo that are raised on the prairie and shot where they graze. The meat is packaged and frozen within about an hour, avoiding the feedlot and slaughterhouse messes that can turn cattle operations into a pathogen nightmare.

Careful meat consumers may also want to study up on a preservative packaging technique involving the counterintuitive deployment of carbon monoxide. These telltale puffy packages pump the gas around the meat, and the treatment can help keep beef looking red and healthy for twenty days on the shelf. The problem is, consumer advocates warn, the meat may still be spoiling under the mask of a better color. The meat industry and regulators worked out one of those head-slapping euphemisms for the process—"modified atmosphere packaging," as if it were just a pine tree air freshener in the family sedan. It may be hard to tell which mainstream packagers use the technique, so look for a "natural" label on the beef. "Natural" packagers can't use carbon monoxide.

As you head toward the produce aisle, remember that the total time from your grocery store cooler to your refrigerator should never be longer than four hours, according to most safety experts. Some say even two hours is pushing it.

The first thing that might hit you in produce is a rainstorm. Ever wonder about those artificial thunderstorms that emanate from hidden speakers and spout a rainforest mist from overhead spigots? Do they actually clean the lettuce? Are they creating a toxic pool of festering bacteria under your green onions? Are they freshening things up or making things worse? Most kitchen advisors call it a draw. The cold water can revive and preserve greens, keeping them from drying out and becoming vulnerable to various forms of rot. But they can also make dessicated greens look more alluring than they deserve. Ignore the distracting rainstorm and use your powers of discrimination to find a fresh sample.

The number-one question here in produce is bruised fruit: in need of a good, understanding home, or dangerous to your happy home? Kitchen scientists are more worried about scratch-and-dent fruit than they used to be, now that they have powerful microscopes and video that can show minute pathogens invading openings at a once invisible level. You might as well get your money's worth and seek out the least blemished fruit. If you do take home some orphaned apples or beat-up pears, cut generously around the bruises and dents that can act as wide-open doors to bacteria.

Bag the produce before putting it in your cart. The plastic can be recycled, and an extra barrier between the greens and the cart, or the fruit and that drippy meat, is another food safety bonus. You don't know where that cart has been—it's fairly likely the germ mobile recently toured the store carrying a sneezy kid eating a sticky fruit roll-up. Keep the bagged produce away from your chicken and other raw meats, even if the meats are also in plastic bags. It only takes a drop of chicken juice dribbling out of the bag to contaminate your veggies. The produce bags have the added bonus of keeping your purchases off the checkout conveyor belt, which just in the last hour has likely hosted everything from fast-thawing ribs to bleach.

There are a few areas and shelves in the grocery store most food safety experts just don't want you near, no matter how careful or lucky you think you are. To name a few:

- the part of the seafood aisle offering oysters from the Gulf of Mexico
- raw—meaning unpasteurized—milk and milk-based products, such as Mexican-style "queso fresco"
- health-food sprouts, from alfalfa to radish to mung bean

The oysters are too often contaminated with dangerous bacteria, especially in summer. Raw milk products are notorious contributors to outbreaks, including one of the deadliest in the modern era. Sprouts contribute up to 40 percent of all produce-related illness cases in a given year, because the time, warmth, and humidity it takes to grow them from seeds are all safe havens for bacteria. If the health food side of you wins when it comes to sprouts, cook them thoroughly instead of eating them raw. Throw them in the stir fry for as long as you cook the other vegetables, and don't just toss them in at the end for a quick sauté.

Natural grocers have one last buying tip for the growing number of consumers looking to nuts as a protein alternative for vegetarians and those cutting back on red meat. Extra-careful stores will refrigerate pistachios, almonds, and other nuts, as leaving them out for too long at room temperature can risk rancidity.

There's one last grocery-store-related step after you've brought it all home. Pleased with yourself because you remembered to use the reusable shopping bags that were drifting aimlessly around your back seat? Great, but don't forget to throw them in the washing machine. Bacteria love to reuse things, too, unless somebody breaks the cycle.

DURING PREPARATION

When unpacking your grocery bags, think about where you are putting things in the refrigerator. Put the most vulnerable foods deep in the fridge, where they will stay the coldest. Don't put eggs in the door, even though some refrigerators are designed with egg trays there. Make sure you store meat on shelves below produce, not on top of it. Restaurants are written up by health inspectors for putting raw meat on shelves above vegetables and fruits that will be served raw because the meat could drip on them. Some experts even suggest storing raw meat not only in a plastic bag, below the vegetables, but also in a plastic container that would collect any leakage.

Thinking about chomping into that apple you just pulled out of the grocery bag and set on your counter? Considering popping a few grapes straight out of the bag and into your mouth? Hang on. Don't assume the produce you buy at the supermarket, even the shiny, red delicious apples or the pretty, rosy nectarines, are ready to eat. Tempting as it is to bite right in, wash the apple first. The majority of experts we talked to advised scrubbing produce with a brush and water—just tap water. Not soap and water. Not even one of those sprays sold in the produce section at the grocery store that claims to remove wax, germs, and pesticides. The truth is that studies have shown the sprays don't work any better than plain old tap water. And soap film clings to your food. Not very appetizing.

If you don't have one, invest a few dollars in a produce scrub brush. It's similar to a potato scrubber or those bristled brushes used to wash dishes. Just before you're going to eat a piece of fruit or a veggie, hold it under tap water and scrub it. This will help remove any dirt and bacteria lurking on the surface. As for fruits with a rind or peel, experts recommend scrubbing those, too, if you're planning to cut into them, which could drag any bacteria clinging to the peel or rind into the center of the fruit. It may sound over the top to rinse off a banana before you eat it, but if you're going to slice it in half and save part for later, or hand half to each of your kids, wash it first. Also, it's best to wash produce right before you're going to eat it. Otherwise, whatever bacteria you didn't remove during that tap-water bath is going to multiply as it sits on your counter or in a baggie in the refrigerator. *Listeria* is one of the bacteria that thrive even in the cool temperatures of a refrigerator. That's something to keep in mind if you're thinking of assembling a fruit salad from a bunch of half portions sitting as leftovers in your fridge for the past few days. Experts advise against saving half a piece of fruit. Better to toss that half an apple that's been hanging out in the refrigerator, growing bacteria, than repurpose it for a salad or sneak it into a lunch box.

Keep in mind, though, that if certain produce is contaminated at the farm or on the truck on the way to the grocery store, there likely isn't a lot consumers can do at home to mitigate that. Consider the surface of a strawberry, with all its nooks and crannies around the seeds. It's nearly impossible to scrub out any lingering bacteria without demolishing the berry.

Even though it won't work on a delicate strawberry, keep your produce scrubber handy for other fruits, everything from pears to zucchini. And just as you should throw your reusable grocery sacks in the laundry every once in a while, make sure you stick your produce scrubber in the dishwasher about once a week.

As for other kitchen gadgets on the market that promise to protect you from bacteria, don't get carried away. Antibacterial cutting boards are kind of silly, according to our experts, who doubt they actually work. Instead, use common sense and make sure not to cut vegetables on the same cutting board you just used for raw meat, unless you disinfect it first with hot water and soap. One expert put antibacterial cutting boards in the same category with many other antibacterial products that have become all the rage—a special coating can't protect you from a careless, easily avoided move. Not only can antibacterial materials kill healthy "background" organisms, they can give a false sense of security. Just because your car has antilock brakes doesn't mean you should drive as fast as you want—an antibacterial surface can't make up for other food safety mistakes.

There's no need to scrub all the carrots, celery, and potatoes you are about to toss into the crockpot. Just give them a quick rinse to remove dirt; cooking is going to kill any dangerous pathogens hanging out on the vegetables. If you are planning on eating produce raw, wash it. The salad you're planning to serve, tossed with baby spinach and spring greens? The mist sprinkling on it every few minutes at the grocery store doesn't suffice. Wash your lettuce with tap water, then pat it dry and let it air out a few minutes on your clean counter. Here's the exception: if you buy packaged, prewashed lettuce in a bag, don't take it out and wash it again. Experts say the lettuce will stay cleaner if you transfer it directly from bag to bowl instead of running it through the sink and letting it lie on the counter. Never prepare a bath for your lettuce in the kitchen sink, letting it float around in there. You might think you're making it cleaner, but more likely, you've just contaminated it with bacteria that was lurking in the sink.

For the same reasons, use separate cutting boards and cutting utensils for produce and meat. At the least, wash the cutting boards in a sanitizing solution before switching uses. Some food experts have given up on the debate between plastic or wooden cutting boards; the plastic boards are easier to throw into the dishwasher for a good "sanitizing" cycle, but they can accumulate many of the same deep grooves and abrasions as a wooden board. The current wisdom is to sanitize all kinds of boards frequently, and toss out old cutting boards more often than you're used to. If the wooden ones have been through the washer so many times their glue seams have fallen apart, then it's time to use them for kindling anyway. Never chop green salad onions atop the board where you just finished tenderizing a raw pork chop.

One of the great kitchen debates is whether you should rinse meat before you cook it. Most experts say no. It's true running raw chicken under water is going to rinse off some *Salmonella* or *Camphylobacter*, but it's also true that you've just increased the odds you're going to drip some of the chicken juice on your counter, maybe even the floor. Not to mention your sink where you are placing other dishes and utensils. There is less chance for contamination if you take the chicken out of the package and head straight for the cutting board or frying pan. A splatter of bacteria-laden turkey juice, for example, can land six feet away, according to the Center for Science in the Public Interest. Six feet. If you cook it properly, any harmful bacteria will die.

DURING COOKING

So now you're actually cooking, and there's nothing left to worry about but making sure the pasta is al dente and stirring the mushrooms so they don't burn, right?

Almost. We're trying to avoid words like *worry* when you're finally in the kitchen and nurturing your family or friends with a well-planned meal. The world's kitchen safety experts don't want to scare you away from the place; instead they want you to absorb some of the easier food safety rules so that it all feels as natural as honey on biscuits. Now that the produce is chopped and the sauté pans are warming, keep a few simple dos and don'ts in mind while you craft anything from a ham and cheese to a Beef Wellington.

Do keep washing your hands frequently, as you go back and forth from browning chicken to assembling a berry-nut salad. Just as you want to keep a dripping bag of raw chicken breasts well below or away from a head of red leaf lettuce, you want sanitary hands to be the barrier between handling meat and sorting greens that are going to be eaten raw.

This next advice may seem obvious: Don't cook when you're sick. But washing hands and wearing gloves in a restaurant kitchen seems obvious, too, and look how many employees don't do that—more than 50 percent, in one recent study. Don't be the one to spread strep through the whole family. You may think you're good about sneezing into your elbow, like the health department cartoons show, but just beyond your elbow is a plate of sliced pears. It's very hard to make your hand washing keep up with your unconscious series of touches to the nose, the eyes, the mouth—all places where germs are weeping at an alarming rate. Call for take-out. Or get your spouse or one of the kids to open a can of soup.

The best thing you can do, that few cooks have learned yet, is to get a good meat thermometer and learn how to use it properly. Many cooking stores or websites offer handy fridge magnets with the safe internal heat temperatures for a variety of meats. Slap it on the fridge next to your kid's spelling test. As Ohio State's Lydia Madeiros puts it, most families remember they have a meat thermometer on only one day of the year: Thanksgiving, when mothers-in-law are expert at sowing doubts about how much heat has penetrated a stuffed turkey. Cooks may have been misled by extensive discussions about *E. coli* in ground beef, thinking that large muscle meats like roasts or whole hams are safer because a lesser-cooked interior has not been exposed to dangerous pathogens in the way an enormous vat of ground beef pieces has. The principle may be true, Madeiros points out, but the safest method is to have all parts of the meat reach at least the minimum temperature. Just as in cantaloupe and other produce, carving and slicing brings any contaminants on the exterior of meat right through to the middle, and from the middle out the other side. Meeting the minimum temperature erases that concern. Use the thermometer in casserole dishes, too, the experts add. The interior of any mixture needs to meet the minimum for the most dangerous element in the mix.

Whole cuts of beef, lamb, pork, and veal should be cooked to at least 145 degrees internal temperature, measured with a thermometer. Consumer preference may go higher than that, to well-well done, but 145 degrees is the minimum safety threshold.

Ground meats, whether beef, lamb, or pork, should be cooked to at least 160 degrees. Ground meats can be more dangerous because the grinder has taken surface bacteria into the middle, harder to reach with heat, and because grinders can mix in batches of meat from multiple sources.

Poultry products should be cooked to a minimum of 165 degrees, with the thermometer piercing the thickest portion of the breast or the innermost section of the thigh and wing.

This also may seem obvious, but many a picnic goer has watched in horror as their host took cooked chicken off the grill and stacked it on the same unwashed plate that carried the raw chicken out to the barbecue. That's a recipe for disaster, and a good justification for sending your teenagers out to get well-cooked replacement tacos. Change or wash all cooking utensils and plates between the raw-meat stage and handling of the final product.

The heat standard also applies, surprisingly, to meats you thought someone else has already cooked for you. Deli meat packages can say "precooked," but *Listeria* in particular loves to hitchhike from the deli processor to those sliding drawers in your fridge. The sliced deli meat can suffer a multiplication of bacteria in the *Listeria*-friendly chill of the refrigerator. Sliced ham, beef, and turkey should ideally be heated in the oven to the recommended minimums for meats before serving in sandwiches, especially for the elderly, pregnant women, and anyone with a compromised immune system from a previous illness. More simple: zap them in the microwave until steaming. If that seems unlikely to make its way into your kitchen routine, consider buying sliced meat made with an antibacterial in the packaging.

If it's cookie dough or cake batter you're whipping up, do not dip a finger in and taste while the eggs are still raw. Yes, your children think it's a crime to let cookie dough go unsampled before it hits the oven. Tell them that the bathrooms and sick beds of many a Toll House were overrun by extremely unhappy customers who downed some bacteria with their tasty, raw dough. If you must, simply must have some egg-based foods in their uncooked state, you'll have to do some extra legwork ahead of time. Pasteurized egg-replacement products in milk-carton-like containers sit in all grocery store coolers near the dairy, and they taste fine when mixed with other ingredients. And there are supplies of eggs pasteurized in the shell if you look hard enough, starting with the customer service desk at your local grocery store. They can place special orders when they see some demand.

While your kitchen becomes a symphony of good smells, keep an eye on how long this is all taking. If something's not getting used for a long time, either as meal prep or as a leftover, get it back in the fridge or freezer. Consumer advocates say food can sit out safely about two hours at room temperature before excessive bacteria growth begins; at ninety degrees on a hot day or an outdoor party, food should be stored after an hour. "Outbreaks are often from temperature abuse," said one food scientist.

CLEANUP AND LEFTOVERS

Here is a recipe so simple you can memorize it right now: add one tablespoon of bleach to one gallon of water. Done.

Mix up a spray bottle of this solution from time to time and keep it under your sink. Use it on your countertops, cabinet handles, and the shelves of your refrigerator every once in a while to disinfect what was left behind by leaky to-go containers, last week's leftovers you forgot to throw away, and the chocolate milk carton your kid insisted on saving and then forgot within ten minutes.

The bleach solution works well, too, for cleaning out your sink. Just fill your sink with water and add the right number of tablespoons, depending on how many gallons it holds. Of course, if you'd rather not bother with making your own cleaning solution, a store-bought one also works.

No reason to act hysterically with the bleach. Most of the time, a simple wipedown of the countertops with a clean, wet cloth after you've finished cooking will do the trick. Best to make a daily habit of tossing yesterday's washcloth into the laundry basket and grabbing a fresh one. If you've splashed chicken juice on the counter, though, or set eggshells down after you've cracked them into your pancake mix, reach for the disinfectant. That way, when you put your fresh pear on the counter later, it's not going to sit on *Salmonella*.

Another good habit: put cutting boards, sink sponges, and lunch boxes in the dishwasher occasionally on the "sanitize" or "antibacterial" cycle. And as we've said before, if your cutting board is deeply rutted or damaged, offering pathogens a safe place to hang out and grow, throw it away.

A 2013 "swab study" uncovered some forgotten corners of the kitchen that cleanliness aficionados might want to adopt for their next weekend project. The National Science Foundation (NSF) International Household Germ Study asked twenty families to swab fourteen common items in their kitchens, and then turn in the samples to see what would grow in a petri dish. They sought growth of *E. coli*, *Salmonella*, and *Listeria*, among other undesirables.

The worst five locations turned out to be the fruit and vegetable drawers in refrigerators, the rubber gasket where your blender jar meets the base motor, can openers, and rubber spatulas. The study recommended a few fixes most cooks wouldn't think of: remove the produce and meat drawers from the fridge entirely, and wash with mild detergent, or a solution of one tablespoon baking soda in a quart of warm water. For blenders, disassemble as much as the design allows, down to separating the gasket on both sides if possible. Then toss it in the dishwasher if made for that, or rinse in hot, soapy water and allow to dry before reassembling. Can openers—imagine how many times the rollers have hit and absorbed tuna juices—should be tossed in the dishwasher; and if your spatula comes apart, break it up and clean both ends, with extra scrubbing for the nooks where the handle fits into the rubber or metal blade.

As for the leftovers in your refrigerator, do you wonder how long you can save the manicotti you brought home from your favorite Italian restaurant? How long is too long to keep the rest of the macaroni and cheese your kids had for lunch today? Should you even bother to put sushi in the refrigerator if you don't finish it all at dinner—or should you just throw it away?

Your grandmother might tell you to keep leftovers for a week. You've likely heard of families that have leftover night once a week, where everything that didn't get eaten all week is set out for one final smorgasbord. But evolving wisdom on food safety says a week is too long to keep many kinds of leftovers. Advisers are becoming more conservative about how long food should hang around in the refrigerator. Two to four days is the limit—two days for more perishable foods, such as Hollandaise sauce; four days for pasta. Ohio State actually now tells consumers not to hold leftovers more than three days, after decades of public health inspector codes using seven days as the standard. "That's controversial," Ohio State's Medeiros acknowledged. But she is unapologetic. "Plan to eat your food. Don't plan to have it sitting around forever."

The sushi? Don't even save it. "You enjoy it and you throw it away," says Sarah Klein with the Center for Science in the Public Interest.

As for cut fruit, don't save it longer than a day.

Never save anything in an open aluminum can, like soup or the refried beans from burrito night. Put leftovers in an airtight container to limit bacteria growth. And when putting away warm leftovers, use shallow containers, no more than two inches deep. If the container is any deeper, the food will not cool fast enough to slow growth of some forms of bacteria.

Check your refrigerator every once in a while to make sure it is no warmer than forty degrees Fahrenheit. Your freezer should remain below zero. For the majority of foods, temperatures hotter than 135 degrees or colder than 41 degrees stop most bacteria growth.

Remember, bad food doesn't always show signs it's gone bad. In doubt? Throw it out.

QUICK TIPS LIST

At the grocery store:

- Shop for dry goods first, cold items and produce later. Try to keep your total time from grocery store to refrigerator close to two hours, and never more than four hours.
- Put packaged raw meat in a plastic bag.
- Don't buy dented cans.
- Don't buy bruised fruit, unless you're planning to cut off the bruised part and well around it.
- Wash your reusable grocery bags every couple of weeks.

Preparing the meal:

- Buy a produce scrubber and use it on fruits and veggies, especially the ones you are going to eat raw.

- Put the scrubber in the dishwasher every week or so.
- Wash melons, bananas, and other fruits with a peel if you are planning to slice through them with a knife.
- Wash produce right before you eat it, not when you unpack your groceries.
- Don't wash prewashed lettuce.
- Don't fill your sink with water and let lettuce float around in it to "clean it."
- Don't rinse meat before you cook it.
- Use separate cutting boards and other utensils for produce and meat. Wash and dry between uses.

While cooking:

- Don't prepare food when you are sick.
- Wash your hands frequently.
- Get a good meat thermometer, and learn how to use it.
- Heat packaged deli meat to steaming before eating. *Listeria* lurks in the packaging facilities and isn't deterred by refrigeration.
- Don't leave food out for longer than a couple of hours. To kill bacteria, food should be kept hotter than 135 degrees or cooler than 41 degrees.
- Don't eat raw eggs. If a recipe calls for raw eggs, use either the pasteurized eggs in a carton or ask your grocer to special order eggs pasteurized in the shell.
- Don't use the same platter for raw meat and cooked meat.

Cleanup:

- Wipe down all used surfaces, including the refrigerator, with a clean cloth and, occasionally, a bleach solution.
- Put cutting boards, sink sponges, and scrub brushes in the dishwasher, and use the "sanitize" or "antibacterial" cycle.
- Discard deeply rutted or damaged cutting boards with hiding places for bacteria.
- Eat leftovers within three days and cut fruit within a day.
- At normal temperatures, cooked food can be left on counters about four hours. In temperatures above ninety degrees, put it away within two hours.

7

KILLER SPROUTS AND SLIMY SPINACH: THE MOST DANGEROUS FOODS MAY SURPRISE YOU

Fresh fruits and vegetables, meat, eggs, and fish are the bulk of a healthy grocery list. They are also some of the foods most likely to make you sick. This list of riskiest foods doesn't contain processed chicken nuggets, crackers, or cans of soup, although it's not unheard of for those less-healthy foods to cause foodborne illness. It's the foods that come fresh from animals, or the dirt, that are most likely to contain *E. coli*, *Salmonella*, and other potentially deadly pathogens.

Several food safety institutes, as well as the Centers for Disease Control and Prevention, have published lists of foods considered most risky, foods to worry about but not necessarily stop serving for dinner. Some of these foods are only now emerging as problems, and it's unlikely the casual grocery shopper, or eater, could name more than two or three. Food fads are evolving everywhere from the grocery store's hot-food bar to the corner bakery to the Internet, where nearly any food or spice is "one click away." Think back to when you were a kid: How often did you eat raw spinach? Now it anchors every salad bar. It's no wonder the plodding machinery of government can't keep up.

The list here is a compilation of research, brought up to date with the latest foodborne illness outbreaks that have changed the way Americans eat. It doesn't include everything. Berries and peanut butter, which have been linked to several outbreaks, didn't make the cut, for example.

It's not a list of foods people should never eat. It's more like a list of foods that should come with a warning label about foodborne illness. Some of you might choose never to order them again—sprouts maybe, or raw milk, or oysters. Others you should eat with caution, and ideally, well done.

SPROUTS

A little extra something on your sub sandwich to give it a refreshing crunch? Probably wise to just say "no thanks" to sprouts. Eating them isn't worth the risk.

Sprouts are inherently dirty, in fact. The way they are grown makes them prone to contamination, and cleaning them off before eating isn't likely to get rid of those illness-causing germs. Sprout seeds can carry bacteria, typically *Salmonella*, which thrives in the warm, moist growing environment that sprouts crave. Most food-illness experts recommend skipping them altogether, no matter whether they are alfalfa, mung bean, or clover. Even lightly cooked sprouts have been linked to numerous ill-nesses in the last several years.

"I wouldn't touch sprouts. They are just too dangerous," said Sarah Klein, an attorney in the food safety program at the Center for Science in the Public Interest.[1]

The squiggly little veggies that add texture to sandwiches, salads, and many Asian foods have been banned from at least one famous American sub shop because of their multiple links to food outbreaks. Jimmy John's Gourmet Sandwich corporate officials stopped serving sprouts on their sandwiches in 2012. The decision came after the popular chain was as-sociated with an *E. coli* outbreak that spanned eleven states and sickened twenty-nine people[2]—the fifth outbreak involving Jimmy Johns' sprouts since 2008. "Jimmy decided he was tired of the negative press from it and he thinks sprouts aren't necessary for Jimmy John's to rock," franchise owner Will Aubuchon told the *Daily Express* in Kirksville, Missouri.[3]

Other sandwich and salad chains, including Jason's Deli and Erbert and Gerbert's Sandwich Shops, also dropped sprouts, at least temporarily. Jimmy John's had switched to clover sprouts from alfalfa sprouts a couple of years earlier, but the outbreaks continued.

In 2011, the Centers for Disease Control and Prevention linked raw clo-ver sprouts from nine Jimmy John's restaurants to twelve illnesses in five states. A year earlier, one of Jimmy John's suppliers, Sprouters Northwest of Kent, Washington, recalled its clover sprouts because they had been linked to illness in the Pacific Northwest.[4]

Also in 2010, the Illinois health department reported that 140 people were sickened in an outbreak connected to alfalfa sprouts contaminated with *Salmonella*. Many of the victims reported eating at Jimmy John's. The FDA issued a public notice telling people to avoid Tiny Greens brand alfalfa sprouts and spicy sprouts (alfalfa, radish, and clover) from Tiny Greens Organic Farm in Illinois. Federal investigators found *Salmonella* in a water runoff sample collected at the farm.[5]

In 2009, a sprout outbreak—also linked to Jimmy John's—sickened 235.[6] Nebraska health officials knew something was dangerously wrong when they found six cases of *Salmonella* Saintpaul in rapid succession. The sprouts were traced back to sprout-growing centers in a handful of states, all of which had purchased sprout seed from the same Kentucky seed producer. It was the seeds that were contaminated with *Salmonella* bacteria.

Here's one more cautionary story, in case you're not yet convinced. In 2008, sprouts from a Jimmy John's in Boulder, Colorado, contaminated with *E. coli* O157 sickened several University of Colorado students, giving them bloody diarrhea and cramping.[7] In all, twenty-eight people were ill.

Although Jimmy John's saga with sprouts is one of the more high-profile stories, the sub chain clearly isn't the only one that's had trouble with them. Sprouts made the top ten "riskiest foods" list prepared by the Center for Science in the Public Interest because they were linked to thirty-one major outbreaks from 1990 to 2009.[8] The vast majority of those outbreaks were caused by various types of *Salmonella*; a handful were *E. coli*.

Federal officials have recommended since 1999 that children, the elderly, and people with compromised immune systems not eat raw sprouts.[9] Whether or not you fit in that category, you might want to think twice before you reach for the salad bar tongs in the sprout bin.

GROUND TURKEY AND POULTRY

Which is better to feed your kids for lunch: processed chicken nuggets from the freezer section or a burger made from ground turkey? The answer depends on whether you are more worried about feeding the children nitrates, sodium, and saturated fat or reducing the risk of ingesting illness-inducing *Salmonella* or *Campylobacter*.

Poultry was ranked the number-one deadliest food in a 2013 foodborne illness outbreak study by the CDC.[10] *Campylobacter* and *Salmonella* bacteria in turkey and chicken were the number-one and number-four most worrisome causes of foodborne illness in the United States in terms of the seriousness of the disease; the long-term, debilitating effects; and the cost of treatment, according to an extensive analysis of CDC data by the Emerging Pathogens Institute at the University of Florida.

"There is a tendency today to assume that if it's in a nice, sealed, wrapped package at the grocery store, it's sterile," said Dr. Glenn Morris, director of the institute.[11] "It's not. It's covered in *Campylobacter*."

Campylobacter is not something you want to get. In a small percentage of cases, a *Campylobacter* infection leads to the severe, lifelong disease of Guillain-Barré syndrome, a disorder in which the body's immune system attacks itself. The subsequent nerve damage progresses to muscle weakness and paralysis. "We're not talking about just a little bit of diarrhea here," Morris said.

This doesn't mean people should quit eating poultry. It means they should "treat it with respect," Morris advises. Don't cross-contaminate in the kitchen. And cook it, thoroughly. That means 165 degrees on a meat thermometer.

Chicken and turkey rank high on the list of concerns for the CDC, yet the agency often does not differentiate between whole chickens and ground meat when it comes to public reporting. Poultry was the fourth most common food implicated in all outbreaks in 2009 and 2010, according to the CDC's national food surveillance network. However, the agency tracks it simply by "poultry" without further detail about specifically what kind of poultry consumers should fear most.

Cooked improperly, all poultry is dangerous. But ground turkey has had its share of bad news in the last several years, particularly in 2011, when ground turkey contaminated with *Salmonella* Heidelberg sickened 136 people in thirty-four states, killing one person.[12] Cargill Meat Solutions, which has since revamped its safety protocols and added a high-pressure, elevated-temperature water wash that disrupts bacteria cells in ground turkey and "neutralizes" them, recalled thirty-six million pounds of the stuff.[13] That same year, twelve people were struck ill, including three hospitalized, by *Salmonella hadar* in turkey burgers sold at Sam's Club.[14]

Especially worrisome about those outbreaks was that they involved antibiotic-resistant *Salmonella*. The frequency of such outbreaks is rising, causing concern among consumer groups and food scientists. The Center for Science in the Public Interest petitioned the U.S. Department of Agriculture in 2011 to prohibit the sale of poultry or ground meat containing four strains of *Salmonella*. At the end of 2012, the USDA implemented stricter pathogen controls for raw ground turkey and chicken, requiring all manufacturers to update their pathogen control plans.[15] It wasn't as stringent as what consumer advocates had asked for, but it was a sign that federal officials were focusing more attention on contaminated poultry.

Banning any poultry with the four antibiotic-resistant strains of *Salmonella* hasn't been a popular method of cutting down on foodborne illness. Government regulators and meat processors contend that if meat sold in stores contains the bacteria, proper cooking will destroy it and make the food safe to eat.

A federal surveillance program has been tracking antibiotic-resistant bacteria on meat since 2002. Scientists at state health departments across the country purchase chicken, turkey, beef, and pork at local grocery stores to isolate surface bacteria, which is sent to a federal lab. The Center for Science in the Public Interest analyzed data collected through that U.S. FDA program, called the National Antimicrobial Resistance Monitoring System, before petitioning for tougher regulation.[16] While *E. coli* is considered an "adulterant" in beef, *Salmonella* and *Campylobacter* are allowed in chicken as the cost of doing business.

Salmonella that is resistant to commonly prescribed antibiotics is concerning because without effective prescription drugs to treat the illness, there is greater risk of severe health issues and death. Most cases of *Salmonella* poisoning go untreated, but, especially in the very young, the very old, and those with compromised immunity, the bacteria can spread beyond the gut and invade the body. "You have a consumer who becomes ill and goes to the hospital and is told the roster of antibiotics that would normally be used might not be effective or as effective," said Klein, with the Center for Science in the Public Interest.

Relying on consumers to kill the bacteria through cooking isn't a safe policy, some experts have contended. A drop of chicken juice that splashes in your kitchen can land halfway across the room. And most people don't use a meat thermometer to make sure their ground beef reaches the recommended 160 degrees or their ground turkey reaches 165 degrees.

But the American Association of Meat Processors has warned that consumers will pay the price if the USDA declares the four strains of *Salmonella* to be "adulterants," meaning they are a "poisonous or deleterious substance" that makes the meat dangerous to health. "Just declaring something an adulterant doesn't solve the problem," said Jay Wenther, executive director of the association. "That is almost a false sense of security. We try to limit any type of pathogens in the product to begin with, but you can't reduce it down to zero."[17]

If the strains of bacteria are banned from raw meat products, ground meat and poultry carcasses found to contain them would have to be either thrown away or cooked before sale. Until then, which is unlikely to come any time soon given the reluctance of the industry, assume the worst about chicken and cook it to 165 degrees.

DELI MEATS

Many obstetricians tell pregnant women not to eat deli meat, and for good reason. *Listeria*—which can kill a fetus—lurks between slices of oven-roasted turkey and black forest ham.

Deli meat consistently ranks near the top of food science lists of the country's most dangerous foods. *Listeria* bacteria is stubborn; it survives and multiplies even at cold temperatures—including the refrigerated deli and hot dog section at the supermarket. Food scientists call it a "production pathogen," meaning it creeps into a factory, probably on the meat slicing machines, and is difficult to kill off. *Listeria* can contaminate deli meats after the cooking process and before the packaging. "It requires scrupulous attention in a plant to keep *Listeria* out," said Dr. Morris at the University of Florida. "It's a big problem."

The only way to kill *Listeria* is to heat the meat to steaming first, which is a pain and not all that appetizing. Zap it in the microwave before making a sandwich, especially if you are pregnant or have a compromised immune system. On average, about 104 people die each year in this country because their deli meat was contaminated with *Listeria*. Nearly six hundred are so sick they are hospitalized, and thousands more are struck with gastrointestinal illness.[18]

Whether the USDA's zero-tolerance policy for *Listeria* is effective is a source of debate. Zero tolerance sounds like a good thing—if any *Listeria* is found on a sample of deli meat headed out of the factory, the entire lot is not fit for sale and must be destroyed. But here's the problem: the stakes are so high that manufactures avoid doing any testing other than the minimum required. Don't ask, don't have to throw it out, is sometimes the operating procedure. Some in the food industry and the FDA have argued federal regulation should allow for low levels of *Listeria* in certain products so that manufactures would not fear testing.

If you think you are safer standing in line at the deli counter to have turkey or ham sliced while you wait instead of buying pouches of prepackaged meat, you are wrong. Data from the USDA's FSIS shows the risk of contamination is five times higher in meat sliced at the grocery store counter.[19] Once a slicing machine becomes infected, it's nearly impossible to clean. And, say, food scientists, retail grocery stores are less likely to undergo frequent scrutiny from inspectors who would swab slicing machines for bacteria. Without proper sterilization techniques, *Listeria* could hang out on a grocery store slicing machine for days or weeks. In a 2010 study, the USDA's FSIS reported that among illnesses and deaths caused by *Listeria* in deli meat, 83 percent were linked to meat sliced and packaged at the grocery store.[20]

Several deli meat health scares in the late 1990s and early 2000s sparked change. Since then, some manufacturers began adding bacterial growth inhibitors to prepackaged meat.

The CDC has long recommended that older people, children, expectant mothers, and those with compromised immunity avoid deli meats unless they've heated them to steaming first, or more precisely, 165 degrees. The federal agency also recommends throwing them away sooner than most people probably do. Don't keep meat sliced at the grocery store more than three to five days. As for prepackaged meat, keep it for up to two weeks if it's still sealed. But once it's opened, toss it within three to five days. Hot dogs, also prone to *Listeria* contamination, shouldn't be kept longer than a week once the package is opened.

Here's another important tip: don't let the juices from a package of hot dogs or deli meat drip on the kitchen counter. Don't cross-contaminate your kitchen by touching a raw hot dog with the same fork you are about to use for macaroni and cheese. And wash your hands after touching raw hot dogs or making a sandwich.

And if you are a mustard fan, slather it on. A study from Washington State University showed a slight reduction in pathogen growth when meat came in contact with mustard.[21]

RAW MILK

It's all the rage to buy farm-fresh food, to seek out free-range eggs and organic vegetables delivered to the door or grown in the backyard. That's all great—but don't take the back-to-nature way of life all the way to raw milk. It's not worth it.

"Raw milk is horrifically dangerous. I would never advise anyone under any circumstances to drink it," said Klein, with the Center for Science in the Public Interest. Food poisoning due to unpasteurized dairy products is among the top four most common foods linked to outbreaks. An average of eight outbreaks are reported each year, and children are particularly susceptible to severe illness and kidney failure. Nearly 80 percent of all raw milk outbreaks reported to the CDC involve at least one child.

Raw milk—meaning unpasteurized or not heated to kill bacteria—that is contaminated with *E. coli* or *Campylobacter* can cause a healthy child to fall desperately ill within a matter of days.

In 2010, an outbreak traced to a Colorado dairy goat cooperative sickened about thirty people, including two young children. At first, Mary Pierce thought her two-year-old couldn't stop throwing up because she had a typical stomach virus.[22] A few days later, she watched in terror as the lethargic young girl was rushed by helicopter to the Children's Hospital Colorado, her little kidneys shutting down. Then Nicole's five-year-old brother, Aaron, fell ill, following her into the hospital and onto a dialysis machine. The cause of their potentially deadly illness: drinking raw goat's milk from a local dairy. "We were just trying it because my son is allergic to dairy. We're not going near it anymore," Pierce said soon after their recovery.

The two kids spent three weeks in the hospital as doctors worked to get their kidneys functioning again. Nicole and Aaron had been drinking raw goat's milk about two or three months before they were infected with a virulent strain of *E. coli*, O157. The bacteria is found in animal manure and likely got into the milk because manure was near the goats' teats. Pasteurization would have cooked out the danger. The kids developed hemolytic uremic syndrome, which causes blood vessels to break up, become meshed with blood platelets, and then damage filters in the kidneys. Nicole and Aaron were anemic and pale and had almost no kidney function, meaning they were not urinating. They spent weeks on dialysis machines to filter their blood and to regain kidney function.

Mary Pierce and her husband, Mike, did research online before deciding to try raw goat's milk because their son was allergic to pasteurized milk. The parents didn't drink any of the goat's milk. "It was so healthy, I was saving it for them," Mary Pierce said. She knew there was a risk of *E. coli* but figured it was highly unlikely. "It's not worth it," she said. "You can't understand until it's your kid lying in the bed."

Kids younger than five and older people are most susceptible to illness from unpasteurized food, said Alicia Cronquist, the epidemiologist with the Colorado Department of Public Health and Environment who played a key role in solving the *Listeria* cantaloupe outbreak. The vitamins killed during pasteurization—thiamine, B12, and C, to name a few—are present in milk in small amounts in the first place, Cronquist said. Any minuscule vitamin gain is overshadowed by the bacterial risk of raw dairy. "I do not drink raw milk. I don't want to play roulette with my health in that way," she said.

Raw-milk proponents say "cooking" milk destroys not only vitamins and "healthy-gut" bacteria but also the enzymes that help digest milk, which is why people who are lactose intolerant can usually drink it without allergic reaction.

Many states ban the sale of unpasteurized milk, yet they allow people to join a farm co-op and buy raw milk directly from "their" farm. CDC officials said a spike in raw milk outbreaks in recent years is likely due to state laws that make it easier for people to buy the raw product.

It's not just raw milk, but all unpasteurized dairy products that people should avoid. The CDC recommends that certain people—the young, old, pregnant, and immune compromised—avoid any cheese that does not say "made with pasteurized milk." The cheese most often blamed is Mexican-style queso fresco, a white cheese. But other soft, unpasteurized cheeses are also suspect, including feta and brie, which are allowed to be made with raw milk because of the aging process.

LEAFY GREENS

In terms of the sheer number of outbreaks, these guys are number one, and many consumers still have trouble believing it. Leafy greens—spinach, kale, chard, cabbage, endive, baby greens, and the rest of the lettuces—were responsible for 2.1 million illnesses in a decade's worth of tallying by the CDC.[23]

For eighty-seven people involved in those outbreaks, it was fatal.

Here's the problem, to summarize: leafy greens are eaten raw, and, too often, they are dirty. About half of the outbreaks linked to leafy greens from 1998 to 2008 were caused by norovirus, transmitted into salads and sandwiches by food handlers who didn't wash their hands or let greens touch dirty countertops. Many others were due to *E. coli* that landed on spinach during the growing or packaging process, likely because the greens touched manure, wild animals, or contaminated water.

If you buy a package of salad mix or plastic tub of spinach that's been contaminated with *E. coli*, there's not much you can do about it. "Washing pre-washed greens isn't going to remove contamination because the bacteria can actually be inside the leaves and stems. You may even make it worse by contaminating it with stuff from your sink," Klein said.

Food safety experts, though, aren't suggesting people stop eating spinach and salads. For the majority of people, the overall health benefits outweigh the risk. Leafy greens help fight cancer, heart disease, and diabetes. "We should be eating a lot of servings of fruits and vegetables per day," said Dr. Patricia Griffin, chief of enteric diseases at the CDC's epidemiology office.[24]

The year 2006 was a bad one for leafy greens. Bagged baby spinach—the kind you would like to assume has been prewashed and is healthy for you—killed three people and sent more than one hundred to the hospital with *E. coli* poisoning.[25] As people were succumbing to illness in twenty-six states and federal investigators were trying to determine which farm was responsible, the FDA warned Americans not to eat any bagged spinach. That outbreak was traced back to Earthbound Farm.

The same year, the dreaded *E. coli* O157:H7 was found in two other outbreaks traced back to leafy greens. In one major outbreak, iceberg lettuce served by Taco John's sickened more than eighty people in Iowa, Minnesota, and Wisconsin.[26]

Once greens are contaminated with bacteria, it's difficult if not impossible to sterilize them without cooking. A chlorine wash after harvest can reduce some of the pathogens, but it doesn't make greens completely safe—even the "prewashed" kind. Since leafy greens appeared on the FDA's national watch list in 2006,[27] farms have improved safety protocols and the seriousness of outbreaks has declined. Still, leafy greens remain one of the riskiest foods.

Many of the leafy-green outbreaks were linked specifically to spinach, and university researchers have found that spinach is more likely than lettuce to harbor bacteria on its leaves, although the reasons are unclear. Measured by the amount consumed, spinach is more often linked to outbreaks and recalls than lettuce. Think about this the next time you line up in the salad shop lunch line: food researchers have found 1 percent of unprocessed spinach, on average, is contaminated with bacteria. Now think about how often you eat it raw. The odds are in your favor, at least. Eating raw spinach has become much more common in the last several years, its popularity climbing on the praise of nutritionists and raw food enthusiasts. A few decades ago, most people ate spinach cooked, killing any harmful bacteria. "Spinach has a higher likelihood of contamination than what we see with lettuce," said Dr. Michael Doyle, director of the Center for Food Safety at the University of Georgia. "I like spinach. My grandmother made a very good spinach dish. She cooked it with vinegar and bacon. We never thought about eating raw spinach—that was for the rabbits. I avoid raw spinach. I eat it cooked."

Improving the safety of spinach and other greens must happen at the farm because if they are contaminated when they show up in your refrigerator, there is not much to do about it, besides cook it. That said, experts recommend keeping it refrigerated, throwing it away by its expiration date, and washing it to remove any dirt on the leaves. If it's prewashed, however, go ahead and eat it straight out of the bag. Washing it again only increases the chances that the spinach will pick up bacteria in your kitchen sink.

EGGS

Reconsider ordering your eggs sunny side up. Don't eat raw eggs, even if it's just in a little dab of cake batter. Or runny ones. Or eggs that have been sitting under a heat lamp for hours on a buffet table. Eggs contaminated with *Salmonella* inside their shells kill more than thirty people in this country on average each year and sicken an estimated seventy-nine thousand.[28]

In the late 1980s, CDC researchers discovered how it was that thousands of people were becoming ill after eating raw eggs that were clean on the surface of the shell and had no cracks. Hens infected with the bacteria in their ovaries laid eggs that carried *Salmonella enteritidis* on the inside of the shell. One might think the FDA and USDA sprung into action to make sure farmers would no longer be allowed to let contaminated chickens lay contaminated eggs that were killing people. But it was not until 2009—twenty years slipping by as the FDA and USDA pointed fingers at each other—that the federal government instituted the "egg rule."[29]

The rule under President Obama requires egg producers to make sure eggs are not contaminated inside the shell, either through pasteurization or other measures. It also requires refrigeration during storage and transportation.

Half of all egg outbreaks in the last decade originated in restaurants or places where food was served to a crowd, according to research by the Center for Science in the Public Interest. The largest egg outbreaks happened in prisons, where on average, 143 people were sick at once.[30]

The reputation of eggs was severely damaged in 2010 when hundreds of Americans grew ill after eating eggs from Wright County Egg Farm in Iowa. FDA inspectors found *Salmonella* in multiple spots on the farm, and it wasn't hard to see why. Manure was piled four to eight feet high in some places. The hen houses were rampant with rodents and flies, alive and dead. The owners of those egg farms left the business and sold the operations to new companies willing to take on the cleanup of not only the farms but also the reputation of the so-called perfect food.

These days, eggs are refrigerated at supermarkets. But it wasn't that many years ago that they were sold at room temperature. The change was the result of researchers figuring out that any *Salmonella* on the outside or the inside of the egg grows rapidly when it isn't cold. Keep eggs in the coldest parts of the refrigerator, not the door. And if your kids must lick the spoon while mixing a cake, use an egg substitute or an egg in the shell that is pasteurized. Look for cartons labeled pasteurized and with a "P" stamped on each shell. Food safety experts also suggest using a meat thermometer when cooking egg dishes, just to make certain they've reached 160 degrees.

PORK

The same parasite associated with cats and, in particular, kitty litter boxes, lives in improperly cooked pork. It's called toxoplasma gondii, and it's among the deadliest of foodborne diseases.

Toxo, for short, is the "quiet, silent disease that nobody knows about," said Dr. Morris with the University of Florida. The foodborne version is estimated to kill about 330 people in this country every year.[31] It causes miscarriage and severe birth defects that can lead to lifetime disability.

Surprisingly, there is no federal regulation of toxo.

The owners of large swine herds in this country have, fortunately, paid attention to toxo and are testing to make sure it is not present in their herds. There is no requirement by the USDA that they must do this, however. Smaller American operators and those in other countries that ship pork to the United States are less likely to keep up with rigorous testing programs to ensure their meat is safe. South American pork, in particular, has a bad reputation for toxo. Ideally, you would avoid buying South American pork chops and pork roast, but the problem is that they typically aren't slapped with a label that says they are South American.

"You have no idea. You are clueless," Morris said. "You buy it in a sealed, wrapped package and there is no indication of where it comes from. You have to take it on faith."

Highly processed pork, including bacon, is safer than more natural cuts, though less healthy and full of fat and sodium.

The most accurate tests for detecting toxo in slaughtered hogs take several weeks, too long to make them a suitable requirement for meat that is headed to stores for consumption, according to the USDA. Besides, federal officials point out, proper cooking, freezing, irradiation, and processing with enzymes kill toxo in slaughtered swine.

Rarely is death by toxo in pork a front-page news story. That's because the pathogen is not normally associated with widespread outbreak; one person typically falls ill at a time. Also, the health impacts do not manifest for months or even years later.

It's estimated that more than sixty million Americans are walking around with the toxo parasite in their bodies, but only a small percentage of us are susceptible to severe illness and death.[32] Pregnant women are on that list, which is why doctors have long recommended that expectant mothers don't clean the kitty litter box.

Here's the most important message regarding pork: eat it well done. If you're not sure, use a meat thermometer to make sure the thickest part of the meat is at least 145 degrees. Wash your hands after touching raw pork. Disinfect countertops touched by raw pork.

OYSTERS AND FISH

Seafood sickened more than a half-million Americans from 1998 to 2008 and killed ninety-four people.[33] In the category of food that comes from the ocean—or, in many cases, fish farms—tuna and oysters jump out as the most dangerous.

Tuna was linked to nearly 270 outbreaks during a ten-year period.[34] The most common cause was a toxin called scombrotoxin, which comes from decomposition bacteria and continues to grow as a dead fish decays. The toxin is not stopped by freezing, cooking, or smoking. So eat tuna only when it's fresh and hasn't been left out too long in the hot sun. In humans, scombrotoxin causes abdominal cramps, nausea, diarrhea, heart palpitations, and loss of vision.

Many of the outbreaks caused by tuna originated in restaurants, likely because people are more likely to eat fresh tuna in a restaurant than cooking it at home.

In July 2012, 425 people were struck with *Salmonella* poisoning after eating frozen raw yellowfin tuna. The illness was serious enough to send fifty-five people to the hospital, though no one was killed.[35] The frozen tuna was used in restaurants to make sushi, and victims of the food poisoning reported to health officials that they had ordered sushi made of spicy tuna from a Japanese steakhouse, among other restaurants. The outbreak spanned twenty-eight states.

At the opposite end of the popularity scale from leafy greens—which many Americans eat multiple times per week—are oysters, which make up an extremely small percentage of the U.S. diet. Yet they cause way more than their fair share of outbreaks—about two hundred per year. Raw or undercooked oysters can make people sick when they are contaminated with norovirus or *Vibrio*.

Oysters are sometimes harvested in waters contaminated with norovirus, which survives all the way into your intestines if you eat the delicacy raw. In one 2012 outbreak, fourteen people who ate oysters at the same New Orleans restaurant fell ill with norovirus.[36] The outbreak caused health officials to shut down a major oyster harvesting area and recall all oysters from the area.

More dangerous than norovirus is *Vibrio*, a bacteria that causes severe diarrhea and cramps in otherwise healthy people. For those with compromised immune systems, *Vibrio* can infect the bloodstream and cause fever, chills, decreased blood pressure, blistering skin sores, and death. Bloodstream infections are fatal about half of the time. Most cases occur in the Gulf states, which is why some food safety experts advise consumers to avoid oysters raised in the Gulf of Mexico. Nearly all Gulf Coast oysters are contaminated with *Vibrio* in the summer months, when the bacteria is rampant in the waters off Texas, Mississippi, Alabama, and other neighboring states, according to one study.[37] In 2009, *Vibrio* killed ten people who ate raw oysters and severely sickened sixteen others.[38] Oysters from the Atlantic had been considered safer until 2011, when two people fell ill after eating some of the shellfish harvested off the coast of Massachusetts. Several more were sickened by *Vibrio* in 2012, and the cases were linked to Massachusetts oysters. Until 2011, it was thought that the temperature of the Atlantic was too cold for *Vibrio* to survive.

The CDC recommends that people with compromised immunity, especially those with liver disease, avoid raw oysters and other raw shellfish—clams and mussels—altogether. Boil shellfish until the shell pops open—and then boil it for five more minutes. If the shell doesn't open, don't eat it. Don't let juices from raw shellfish drip around the kitchen, and if they do, disinfect.

Only heat kills the bacteria. No matter how sophisticated you are about eating oysters on the half-shell on a bed of ice, you can't tell if they are contaminated by smelling or tasting them. Also, dousing oysters with hot sauce—no matter how spicy—does not kill toxins. Neither does alcohol.

BEEF

Don't eat pink hamburgers. The manure staining a cow's hide sometimes ends up on the outside of the meat during slaughter, and when beef is ground into hamburger, that fecal matter can end up in the burger. Many cattle also have *Salmonella* or *E. coli* bacteria in their guts, which comes with them to the slaughterhouse. And one package of ground hamburger could have come from dozens of different cows, all shipped from feed lots to the same slaughter house and processing plant. Packers buy "trim" from all over the world and grind it into massive, mixed-up batches of beef.

Bad beef sent more than three thousand people to the hospital in this country in a ten-year period and was responsible for the deaths of fifty-five, according to the CDC.[39] Those are scary numbers, although they are far lower than hospitalizations and deaths caused by poultry or pork.

Beef safety has improved dramatically in the United States since the terror brought on by the Jack in the Box scare of 1993, when hundreds were sickened with *E. coli* O157:H7 and four children died. It was a wake-up call: American children died because they ate undercooked hamburgers.

Documents discovered during the investigation revealed that Jack in the Box was undercooking its burgers and had been warned by local health departments and employees.[40] But company officials thought cooking burgers to the required 155 degrees—hot enough to kill harmful bacteria—made the burgers too tough.

In 1994, the USDA banned the sale of raw ground beef found to have *E. coli* O157:H7, meaning packing plants were required to test for it. In 2012, the federal agency added six strains of *E. coli* to the banned list for raw meat.

The tests don't cover every pound of meat sold, but a sample of beef that turns up positive results in recalls or impounding.

Cooking beef properly kills the bacteria. The USDA recommends 160 degrees. Left to sit in temperatures above 40 degrees or below 140 degrees—the "danger zone"—bacteria in the meat multiplies. University studies have found that cooking a burger until it's no longer pink does not necessarily mean it reached 160 degrees, so it's best to use a meat thermometer.

Ground beef is implicated more often in outbreaks than steak. That's because the inside of a steak is considered sterile. The exception is when meat is mechanically tenderized with needles, a process used by some restaurants to improve the cut of meat and, in some cases, infuse it with flavor. In recent years, several outbreaks have been linked to tenderized steak. Problem is, they are rarely advertised as such, so ask the server. If you choose a tenderized steak off a menu, or one that promises the infused flavors of bourbon or mesquite, ask for it well done.

TOMATOES AND PEPPERS, THE VINE VEGETABLES

Salmonella can invade a tomato through its roots, flourishing stubbornly inside the vine-grown fruit. Only cooking is likely to kill it. In the growing process, *Salmonella* bacteria can invade through the plant's roots or flowers, or even tiny cracks on the tomato's skin.

All types of tomatoes—vine ripened, grapes, cherry—have been blamed for food-illness outbreaks across the county. In particular, 2005 and 2006 were rough years, but tomatoes contaminated with *Salmonella* are implicated in illnesses each year.

In 2005 and 2006, tomatoes caused four major outbreaks of *Salmonella*, sickening hundreds of people. One study counted more than thirty outbreaks linked to tomatoes since 1990, about half of them due to *Salmonella*.[41] In 2008, a major food-illness outbreak was initially pinned on tomatoes, and the FDA warned Texas and New Mexico residents to stop eating certain types of raw tomatoes. Federal investigators could not pinpoint a specific type of tomato, but they knew many of the sick had reported eating tomatoes. Or rather, salsa. The investigation took months. In the end, after 1,442 people in forty-three states were ill, the FDA found *Salmonella* on a jalapeño pepper and a Serrano pepper grown in Mexico.[42] Federal investigators also found *Salmonella* in the farm's irrigation water.

More than 280 people were hospitalized.

In December 2011, the FDA announced a recall of fresh, Mexican-grown jalapeño and Serrano chili peppers that tested positive for *Salmonella* and were shipped to stores in California, Texas, Oregon, Washington, and Canada.[43]

Dried peppers aren't exempt from *Salmonella*. In October 2011, a California company recalled 1,800 jars of Su-nun brand crushed red pepper because of possible contamination. Routine testing by the USDA found *Salmonella* in a sample.[44]

Food safety experts aren't suggesting Americans strike tomatoes and peppers—the staples of salad, pizza, and salsa—from their diet. But people with weakened immunity—cancer patients on chemotherapy, for example—should consider avoiding fresh tomatoes and peppers. And restaurants should follow suggested guidelines from the CDC to minimize bacteria transfer during food preparation.

Foodborne illness investigations show tomatoes are likely tainted back at the farm, not in the kitchen. But the way people handle tomatoes could lead to more "germ growth," according to the FDA. Without proper handling, tomatoes with *Salmonella* could contaminate nearby tomatoes.

People should keep fresh produce, especially tomatoes, away from other food. Wash them in running water before eating them, but don't soak them in water. If you save part of a cut tomato, keep it in the refrigerator—but not for longer than a few hours. The FDA also recommends restaurant workers wear gloves when handling tomatoes.

MELONS

The cantaloupe outbreak that killed thirty-three people catapulted melons to a national concern. A year later, *Salmonella* on cantaloupe killed three people in Kentucky and sent ninety-four others to hospitals in various states.[45] The melons' scarred reputation means that some people still walk right past them in the produce section or farmers' market. But melons—cantaloupe, honeydew, and watermelon—have long been on the radar of food safety authorities.

Melons, in fact, are among the most troublesome foods in the produce system.

Cantaloupe and other melons made up 16 percent of all produce-related outbreaks in a twelve-year period studied by the FDA and the CDC. That was before the deadly 2011 outbreak of *Listeria* in Colorado, and the 2012 *Salmonella* outbreak linked to an Indiana farm. Of the 406 incidents of food poisoning in Colorado from 1998 to 2010, cantaloupe or honeydew melon were suspected in eight—putting melon in the top ten foods most often suspected of contamination in that state, behind ground beef, lettuce, chicken, and sushi.

"Cantaloupe has been problematical," said David Gombas, senior vice president for food safety and technology at the United Fresh Produce Association in Washington, D.C.[46]

The pocked surface of a cantaloupe provides plenty of crevices for bacteria to latch on. Food safety experts recommend scrubbing the surface of a cantaloupe with soap and water before slicing through one. That step could help prevent foodborne illness—unless the cantaloupe was contaminated on the inside.

Research suggests the sweet nutrients inside cantaloupes entice pathogens on the surface of the fruit to come inside through tiny nicks or cuts. Irrigation water containing *Salmonella* could contaminate the surface of the melon, and perhaps get inside through openings on the surface, according to research published in the *International Journal of Food Microbiology*.[47] Researchers want to study that question more. If that's the case, washing the cantaloupe's surface isn't going to fix the problem. Scientific opinion varies about whether *Listeria* or *Salmonella* bacteria can enter a melon through its roots.

Experts have called for stricter guidelines regarding irrigation water for produce grown on the ground. The FDA has ordered melon farmers to institute best practices and face inspections. But consumers should remember food production starts in the dirt. "The sobering reality of all of this is our food is not sterile," said Colorado health department microbiologist Hugh Maguire. "It may look great and taste wonderful, but it is not sterile."

8

DANCES WITH DNA, AND
RECONSIDERING RADIATION

Frankenfish. Mock meat. Genetically modified corn flakes. Irradiated radishes. Are they a safer way to feed the world, or the largest experiment in eating ever attempted?

Worries of tomorrow's food come rushing upon us before we've even answered the worries of today. The current state of the food supply clearly has issues enough to give a shopper pause in the grocery aisle. Is there any chicken breast for sale in the store that isn't already contaminated with *Salmonella*? Was that cheese pasteurized properly? Did the cantaloupe farmer use enough chlorine in the sanitary wash before shipping the melon across three states?

While these key questions linger, digital messengers deliver the fears of tomorrow. Borne on a flood of half-read Internet links, hyperventilating cable news shows, and forwarded emails from friends who thought the "maverick" views of some local activist sounded scientific, these ominous changes in food arrive in waves of vague anxiety. Is that plant they altered in a test tube already in my cornbread? That mashup salmon breed we heard about—what was it, the Frankenfish?—is it already swimming toward our favorite sushi bar? Is there some part of a cloned animal in our cheeseburgers, or was that supposed to happen next year?

At the same time, we hear of disturbing gaps in the government's oversight of factory-modified foods. As of early 2011, there were 38,718 items for sale on supermarket shelves. The list of allowed chemical additives in that array of products now reaches more than ten thousand. Guess who decided many of those chemicals are "safe"? The manufacturers, and a trade association panel paid for by manufacturers. More than three thousand of those "safe" substances were deemed so by industry, bypassing a formal government decision.[1]

Parents hear protests against the unknown allergens of genetically modified foods, and they wonder if every child with allergies needs to fear soda with high-fructose corn syrup made from genetically modified corn. Does the fact they once created Dolly the cloned sheep mean there are now space-age, test-tube replicas of other sheep in my lamb chop? Is Quorn that thing made from quinoa, or is it that fungus-based meat substitute that somebody said could be toxic?

Surely someone must be on the lookout, sorting all these new foods for us before they become part of our dinner?

A plethora of government agencies, nonprofit organizations, scientific groups and societies, and independent journalists track the waves of allegedly beneficial changes to the food supply in the United States, not to mention a seemingly formidable international gauntlet including the World Health Organization, various UN branches, and the European Union. Genetic engineering's promoters complain that the thicket of regulators and agitating commentators is so dense it costs them more than $100 million in research to get one modified crop through to market.[2]

Yet those watchdogs are overwhelmed by the quickening pace of technology and lobbying efforts by billion-dollar private corporations demanding the earliest possible payback on their lab investments. A business culture addicted to earnings reports every ninety days doesn't have the patience for long-term, government-sanctioned safety studies that many scientists say are the only legitimate test of how a new food will behave inside human consumers years down the road. The main U.S. safety agencies admit that even if they were inclined to, they don't have the time, people, or money to review each and every food gene alteration in the way they might demand for, say, a new cancer drug. A recent Food and Water Watch study cited an estimate that twenty new food-related products embedded with nanotechnology were arriving on world markets every month. Summing up its own inability to sip from the firehose of nanotech—not to mention genetically engineered crops, cloned animals, or "mock meat"—the FDA said, "Few resources currently exist to assess the risks that would derive to the general population."[3] Not exactly a consumer confidence builder.

For many consumers, when it comes to what we eat, delight in the new has been largely replaced by shock of the "new and improved." We've been falsely reassured too many times by Madison Avenue pseudoscientists in costume white lab coats, smiling through enthusiastic plugs for the pesticide DDT, the stimulating effects of tobacco, the lifesaving properties of asbestos, and countless other endorsements later retracted after damning revelations. Yet a good portion of consumers are also exhausted by the daily-terror approach of modern health writing, where the Monday report on the dangers of caffeine is contradicted by the Tuesday endorsement of coffee, and quickly overridden by the Wednesday warnings about margarine. Perhaps we could try to assess the future of food without celebration or condemnation, but with accurate description.

Here are some of the more important and most complex issues encompassing the confusing intersection of food safety and food technology. From GE canola oil to gene-spliced salmon to nanosilver to (Test) Tubesteak, the final answers may be years or decades in the future, but the challenges are already arriving at the grocery store every day, by the truckload.

GENETICALLY MODIFIED FOODS

The science of splicing or injecting new genes into old foods is thick with the alphabet soup of GEs, GMOs, GMs—and less formal, more insulting terms like Frankenfish or Mutant Food. But they all refer to the same thing—something you've eaten for a long time, wedded by force of science to something that didn't use to live in the same chromosomal neighborhood. One gene of one plant melded to another, a bacteria bonded to a cereal grain gene, a living animal's DNA injected into another's.

So you're not sure about these genetic gymnastics, not eager to tuck into those suspect foods? Far too late. What many Americans don't realize is that they've been eating genetically engineered foods for years now. Commodity experts estimate GE seeds are 70 to 90 percent of the field corn market, meaning that spliced DNA is in everything from breakfast cereal to chips to the high-fructose syrup of soft drinks.[4] The great majority of soybeans and canola oil seeds grown in North America are also from genetically modified plants, with other crops following fast. Many seeds come with multiple GE protections built in, a "triple stack" that will fight off herbicide, boring insects, and rootworm.

Humans have, in fact, been genetically modifying their food for thousands of years, since they first herded the biggest wild goats into the same pen for breeding, or chose the maize seeds for next spring from the largest ears of the fall harvest.[5] Whether or not they knew what they were doing at the time, prehistoric humans selected the traits they needed most in their tenuous food supply and both replicated them and enhanced them. Selection led to crossbreeding, the mating of slightly different breeds within the same species to produce better traits, and then hybrids, mating different species with a goal of even bigger improvements. When mountain miners wanted a strong, smart pack animal that could go all day and never pitch over a cliff, they bred male donkeys with female horses and found themselves a genetically modified mule. Long before new forms of genetic engineering became controversial, vast majorities of modern commodity crops were as much a result of lab work as fieldwork, through painstakingly selected and nurtured hybrid seeds.

The iteration of genetic engineering that worries so many of us now is that forced mating we mentioned earlier: a literal injection of genetic material from one plant species into the genetic heart of another to speed up nature's evolutionary mixing and matching by hundreds of thousands of years. (The same goes for newly engineered animal species, as in the "Frankenfish" salmon that brought together in unlikely matrimony the genetic scraps of an Atlantic salmon, a slimy, bottom-feeding eelpout, and a majestic king salmon.) The Flavr Savr tomato was the first modified produce allowed for sale in the United States, in the mid-1990s, taking a common gene that promoted rot in fruit, flipping it into its "anti" version, and inserting it back into a stock tomato to create a fruit that would last longer on the shelf before ripening to mush.[6]

The tomato of tomorrow never really caught on, in part because of bad press about alleged bad reactions in rodents that later turned out to be incorrect, and in part because the sponsoring company was a science lab and not an expert food marketer.[7] Produce has never really caught on in mass-market genetic engineering, because costs and consumer tastes are too unpredictable for crops with relatively small niches.[8] The cereal grains and factory-ready commodities such as cotton, however, were ripe for further engineering because of their uniform nature and enormous market potential. What if you could insert a gene that tolerated drought into traditional wheat, widely expanding the growing zones in hot spots like Africa or Asia? How about a genetic nutrition-booster injected into a crop like rice that is the life staple for billions of people?

American researchers stuck close to their home markets at first, looking at industrialized U.S. agriculture and adapting the situation at hand to the situation they had created. Chemical and seed giant Monsanto already produced the most popular herbicide, Roundup, for millions of acres of Midwestern crops. Spray the fields before planting, and kill all the weeds.

But what if you could produce a crop seed that could survive a Roundup assault? Then you could spray the herbicide all through the growing season, beating back the weeds that cut deeply into yields. Monsanto found a bacterium that could survive against Roundup, and they inserted it into corn seeds. The company then had massive success selling both the resistant seeds and the chemical herbicide to farmers wanting an edge.[9] The concept led the company to dominate the market in a way that left critics in awe of the audacious strategy even as they decried the results. At the same time, other researchers were injecting seeds with extra genes that naturally produced an insect-killing toxin, turning the seeds into a crop-and-pesticide combo in every plant, referred to as Bt. Both the Roundup Ready seeds and the Bt seeds received government approval in the 1990s, and they overwhelmed the market.[10]

The alleged virtues of GE or modified crops are manifold: They grow more food on less land by reducing the yield lost to weeds and pests; they lower the amounts of potentially dangerous pesticides needed to beat back insects; some varieties need less fertilizer because they produce their own, saving costs for marginal farmers and reducing water-polluting runoff; nutritious gene combinations can turn a staid crop into a vitamin pill; and future drought-resistant combinations may soften the damage of global warming.

But what do they do to your body? It's not natural to consume a soup of mix-and-match genes, is it? If we put future food into our present bodies, isn't that both an evolutionary and existential disaster?

So far, the strongest argument against the safety of consumed, genetically modified foods is that they were not studied long enough before taking over store shelves. Actual, proven harm to individual consumers does not yet exist.[11] Opponents, including many credible scientific and environmental groups with a history of responsibly compiling research, have raised potential flags regarding how human digestive systems will handle spliced genes from species never before in our diet. They have also pointed to allergy concerns, and the dangers of a food item that appears to be soy, for example, but which may contain a hidden gene that's toxic for certain users.[12]

As the two-decade mark of mass GE consumption approaches, those fears are not realized.[13] Occasional studies claiming a tangible impact of GE foods on lab animals have been subsequently discredited by a wide range of scientists.[14] No specific allergy issues have arisen, and many commentators have mentioned how hard it would be to sort new allergies from old in a nation where millions are already affected by peanut allergies, and many mainstream foods already held allergic dangers for various subgroups.

A countervailing group of mainstream scientific bodies, from the World Health Organization to the National Academy of Sciences to the American Association for the Advancement of Science,[15] have conducted wide-ranging literature reviews and GE assessments, and they declared them no more a threat than traditional food sources.

Those trying to slow down GE foods are frustrated by the food safety questions. Commerce has rushed ahead without scientific proof of safety, they say, and we don't know what we don't know—because GE foods do not have to be labeled as such (a wider-ranging controversy we will revisit in a few pages), people have no idea they've been part of the largest eating experiment of all time. How could they identify a health effect of a substance when they have no idea they are ingesting it?

"With a drug, people know they are taking that drug," said Patty Lovera, a modified foods expert with Food and Water Watch. "We've missed that opportunity to even see if there are health changes fifteen years in, because we don't know what people are eating."[16] Because the FDA's resources in modified foods are so limited, they have thrown up their hands since the first rounds of GE seeds won approval, Lovera argues. Each new filing for a modified food source refers extensively back to the first one approved, building on the same shaky foundation. A good portion of university agriculture and food research, meanwhile, is sponsored by the same corporations profiting from modifications. Independent researchers are not allowed to buy patented seeds for scrutiny, and when someone does dare question the science, "they hit that researcher with a ton of bricks," she said. Lovera noted instances where companies have demanded to review university researchers' work before publication, or where professors have suffered tenure battles after research raising new issues about modified seeds.[17, 18]

There is not a good scientific case against all GE foods, or even against most of them, said Doug Gurian-Sherman, a senior scientist for food and environmental issues with the Union of Concerned Scientists. The point is that even if the first ninety-nine approved GE foods prove safe, there won't be a way of finding the dangerous one-hundredth because no long-term testing is required, and weak U.S. regulators turn much of the review into a voluntary system, he said. "We should not be paranoid about this," he said. But at the same time, "I should not have to guess."[19]

The stronger objections to GE foods involve issues of long-term environmental and agricultural impact and socioeconomic fairness, not the immediate safety of the food itself.

The socioeconomic objections center on GE expanding the corporate-controlled monoculture of American farming and food. Because GE foods take millions of dollars to develop and are then locked up in airtight patents by the corporations who sell them, only enormous farms with satellite-controlled tractors and chemical tanks grouped like high rises can afford to plant them. Big Agribusiness dominates the crops, then with its accumulating cash stores dominates Congress and any regulators who would dare to raise questions. Once planted en masse, environmentalists worry crop traits and matched herbicides will spill over into nearby organic fields or small-farm operations, turning the whole world GE under clouds of gene-modified pollen. U.S. agribusiness will wield even more power when developing nations come calling for modernized agriculture, protecting their prices with GE patents and squeezing out efforts for indigenous, locavore food culture. "It drives diversity out of the food supply, which is not smart in a climate that gets crazier every year," summed up Food and Water Watch's Lovera.

GE promises all sorts of cuts to pesticide and herbicide chemical use, but it produces the opposite effect, opponents add. Weeds sprayed over and over again with Roundup and other herbicides eventually mutate "superweeds" that can resist the chemical assault.[20] Those superweeds are already appearing and multiplying in fields planted with Roundup Ready GE seeds. Scientists are now developing other GE modified seeds that can resist even stronger chemicals, including one called "2, 4-D," tagged fairly or unfairly as one of the components in the notorious Vietnam defoliant Agent Orange.[21] (The most toxic substance in Agent Orange was a dioxin contaminant with another name.) More chemicals spraying around the world also means more exposure to farm workers on the corporate giants' spreads, in addition to any farmers and rural residents living nearby. Taken together, the objections paint a picture of the food powers favoring centralization and corporate science, when a good portion of consumers are heading in the other direction, toward backyard chickens, organic vegetables, and getting to know the local farmer who grew their tomatoes.

Genetic engineering's proponents like to counter those disturbing uncertainties with disturbing certainties.

Just as climate change threatens to scorch some long-fertile areas and drown others, economic development in Asia, Latin America, and soon, Africa, is lifting hundreds of millions of consumers to income levels where they can afford more calories. They want access to the same commodities, from corn flakes to beef steak to tofu, that Westerners have enjoyed for a century now.[22] A British activist who led much of the charge against GE foods in their first years made a highly publicized about-face in 2012, with this mea culpa at the core of his reversal: in less than four decades, the world will have 9.5 billion people and will demand a 100 percent increase in food production from current levels. Organic techniques favored by foodies, Mark Lynas added, often yield only half the crops produced by much-reviled agribusiness farming. "Over a decade and a half with three trillion GM meals eaten, there has never been a single substantiated case of harm," Lynas said, in his oft-circulated speech apologizing for previous opposition to food technology. "The risk today is not that anyone will be harmed by GM food," Lynas went on, "but that millions will be harmed by not having enough food, because a vocal minority of people in rich countries want their meals to be what they consider natural."[23]

GE skeptics who used to be aligned with Lynas, facing the reality of a GE-dominated food stream and the absence of immediate harm, have turned their efforts to universal labeling.[24] You're going to splice new genes into old foods, whether we like it or not? Fine. Tell us when you're doing it, right there on the package and on the menu, so we can make the ultimate capitalist gesture of choosing with our wallet.

After years of battles on the federal and local level, the labeling issue may finally be headed toward a rational compromise. And that's good for consumers, across the spectrum of worry about GE and food safety.

The FDA has so far declined to require labels on GE foods. European government agencies have effectively halted the spread of GE foods across the sea by requiring labels, which food companies have until recently considered a kiss of death for their packaging.[25] Agribusiness and its proponents in university science have long argued that since the GE crop staples are indistinguishable in nutritional value or health effects from traditional foods, labeling will only confuse and worry the consumer. "You can scare people in 30 seconds, but I can't educate them that fast," said a Penn State farm scientist. They get backing from a significant group of academy-level researchers as well, including a 2012 letter from the American Association for the Advancement of Science that reads like a papal directive: In the absence of any evidence of harm, no matter how hard people look, "legally mandating such a label can only serve to mislead and falsely alarm consumers."[26]

There are dissenters, and their influence appears to be growing rather than waning even as millions more GE-modified meals are eaten every day. The AAAS letter prompted an official protest signed by twenty-one doctors and scientists, saying the "Orwellian" dismissal of labeling "tramples the rights of consumers to make informed choices."[27] The right to know is a basic human right, the dissenters said. California's Proposition 37 in 2012 was the first of many statewide efforts to mandate labeling where the FDA and other federal agencies won't. It failed, but closely enough to be a tantalizing rallying cry for future efforts.[28] The prolabeling groups accused the seed, chemical, and food companies of buying votes with corporate media campaigns, while defenders of GE said there was just as much self-interest in the ad campaigns backed by large organic food concerns. Compromises will likely rule the day. "It's just so obvious—even if you love the technology, why shouldn't they tell you what's in there?" asked Patty Lovera of Food and Water Watch. Following a narrow defeat of labeling in California, major food-related companies such as Walmart, Coca-Cola, and Pepsi–Frito Lay started meeting in 2013 with labeling proponents and the FDA, seeking a national labeling standard.[29] It will be hard for the seed companies to resist if the conglomerates that purvey their GE food to the public come out in favor of a national label. The final protest of the laboratories is that silly, easily frightened consumers won't know what to make of it if a bag of Fritos says "May Contain Genetically Modified Materials." That may be true. Yet many labels already use words like *maltodextrin* that very few people stop to understand. And still they buy.

The labeling fight will intensify in coming years as genetic engineering moves past commodity crops and on to animals used for food. For those battles, environmentalists and natural food advocates have much more muscle on their side in the form of furious congressional members from frontline states. If you're planning to make the first GE animal unleashed onto the public a double-modified salmon, you can expect to hear from an Alaskan delegation that retains a grizzly bear's sense of diplomatic justice. When various interests ignore her efforts to block modified salmon, Alaskan Republican senator Lisa Murkowski tells them they can look forward to a visit from her to "discuss Frankenfish."[30]

Frankenfish is the scathingly dismissive name for a swimmer created by the AquAdvantage corporation. It just happens to be the nearest to market of dozens of modified fish species, which mix catfish, striped bass, or flounder with genes from other fish, mice, "or even human beings," the Center for Food Safety warned.[31] Chinook or king salmon genes spliced into a traditional Atlantic salmon allow it to grow twice as big, while cold-water, bottom-feeding eelpout genes push the salmon to feed and therefore grow year-round. The resulting fish would allow farming operations to get hefty specimens to market twice as fast as other salmon.[32]

The AquAdvantage salmon seems like a boon to overfished oceans in an era where fast-developing nations rapidly catch up to Western countries in their taste for seafood as nutritious protein. Twice the fish in half the time—isn't that a formula to save the world?

Loosing that fish upon the oceans terrifies opponents even more than modified crops, which are too far gone to stop. Voracious, dominant GE salmon will escape leaky industrial fish farms and breed their way through the world's oceans, threatening the extinction of the original Atlantic species, objecting scientists have concluded.[33] Fast-growing GE salmon crowded into onshore pens will be so stressed they'll require antibiotics to stay healthy, and human consumption of the antibiotic-permeated flesh will exacerbate drug resistance problems, they add. AquAdvantage, which has tried to bring the fish to market for years, says the fish eggs will be sterile so any escaped GE salmon can't reproduce, and that the adult fish won't ever touch the ocean.

Fanciers of "funny fish"? Get reacquainted with the Alaska delegation.

"You keep those damn fish out of my waters," Representative Don Young (R-Alaska) told the *Washington Post*. "It will ruin what I think is one of the finest products in the world." Of the AquAdvantage corporate parent, Young said, "I can break that company."[34]

While not giving an inch on any of their other objections, food safety advocates say if all else fails they will still demand labeling for any modified fish or subsequent engineered food animals. "Should FDA decide to approve the AquAdvantage GE salmon despite our opposition, clear, mandatory labeling is an absolute must to allow consumers to make informed decisions," the Center for Food Safety wrote.[35] Again, the argument seems more than fair. The best argument against labeling GE corn is that once it's in your cornflake, there's no way to ever distinguish it from any other ear of corn ever grown. But the super-salmon is a bigger threat, producing a big fish never before seen, which could eventually become the GE whale in every ocean. The least we should know is what exactly it is that we're throwing on the grill.

CLONING

Cloned animals should be far less of a food safety concern for American consumers in coming years. Not because the food industry hasn't tried, but in large part because the economics of the god-playing science haven't worked out as planned.

From the purest food safety standpoint, a "cloned animal issue" doesn't exist. The clone is an exact replica of the copied animal, by definition down to the very DNA. Food safety for that new animal is only as good, or as bad, as in the original animal.[36] A steer cloned for beef must still be slaughtered and packaged properly to avoid *E. coli* contamination; it has no advantage or disadvantage over the original.

The operating assumption for years in cloning science was that labs would be able to produce such perfect food animals, whether all-star milk cows or best-bacon fattened hogs, that old breeding methods would be cheaply and thankfully replaced. Every steak would be top choice, every egg grade double-A. Researchers have begun adding in fatty-acid producing traits from earthworms, of all creatures, to farmyard animals, and then cloning those to a new level of alphabet soup: G(enetically) E(ngineered) C(lone). But a funny and disturbing thing happened on the way to the farmyard. Embryos that seemed perfect in the petri dish just wouldn't cooperate months later when leaving the mother animal's womb. A high percentage of cloned animals falter after birth, with defects or abnormally short lifespans, for reasons science hasn't completely explained.

The FDA declared cloned meat and milk safe for eating in 2008, but very little has reached the food supply.[37] The expense of producing enough survivable, full-fledged clones makes the technique incompatible with the factory-farming scale of American beef cattle, hog farming, or chicken warehouses. Artificial insemination, though, allows clone offspring to dominate certain kinds of breeding. Companies specializing in the top agricultural sires select and copy those with the best traits, then ship vials of semen around the world to be "mated" with conventional mother animals. A Penn State animal expert estimates the great majority of U.S. Holsteins—the most popular breed of dairy cattle—are the offspring of just fifty bulls.[38] Clearly, whether cloning catches on or not, we have radically wrenched control of the farm gene pool from "natural" sources.

The few cloned or cloned-offspring cattle, hogs, and other animals do grow old and go out of useful farm service. The FDA asked farmers and ranchers to voluntarily keep such animals out of the human food supply, but that was long before the FDA itself reviewed the science and declared cloned food to be safe for consumption. Aged-out clones do end up in our food, even if in infinitesimal portions. That's why most food activists and consumer groups have once again demanded labeling for any foods that contain cloned stock. They've had no more luck there than in other labeling fights—the FDA said since no one could tell the food apart on a molecular level, there's no reason and therefore no rule to label.[39]

IRRADIATION

There's another potentially game-changing food production technology that you won't have to worry about much in the near future. But be careful what you hope against—this particular technology, which has been "the future of food" on and off for decades now, could be preventing major illness and saving hundreds of lives a year if implemented today.[40] Irradiation's pariah status can be blamed as much on intransigent consumers and opportunistic food activists as it can on any problems with the actual science.

Food irradiation, according to the CDC's chief epidemiologist for food-borne diseases, could stop close to a million infections, 8,500 hospitalizations, and 350 deaths each year even if only half the beef, pork, and poultry in the United States were treated before shipping.[41] With more and more national pathogen outbreaks coming on the green produce side of the food ledger, imagine how many more illnesses could be stopped by existing irradiation technology applied to fruits and vegetables. Frustrated epidemiologists and farm economy experts have two words to describe ongoing opposition to irradiation: "a tragedy," as Penn State's Terry Etherton puts it.

"We must begin to use food irradiation if we are really to make a difference in food safety," argues Michael Osterholm, of the Center for Infectious Disease Research at the University of Minnesota School of Public Health, echoing many of his colleagues.[42] It's an argument that for years has had the official stamp of approval, if not much public relations support, from the FDA.

So why is only 1 percent of the current meat supply irradiated before consumption? And perhaps an even smaller percentage of produce? Because the industry is convinced you as the consumer can't stand the idea, whether or not you actually understand it, and you are not willing to change your mind.

Irradiating food does not mean sticking it in a nuclear reactor core and raising the control rods. It uses one of three different technologies to focus existing particle energy onto food, bumping out free radicals that then kill the DNA of bacterial pathogens such as *E. coli* and *Salmonella*. Viruses like norovirus take higher, potentially aesthetic-damaging levels of irradiation to kill, and they are not usually part of the debate. Proponents liken the process to any other outside force used to change the state of food, whether a microwave for warming, pickling for preserving, or freezing for storage. No "radiation" lingers inside treated food; only one of the processes even uses radioactive material to generate the ionizing energy, and none of that material goes anywhere near the food.[43]

The FDA and many other national and international agencies have reviewed all existing science on what irradiation does to food, looking for signs of harm to the end consumer. They haven't found any. Environmental groups say the free radicals produced "could" affect the food in unknown ways, but scientific analysis of the nutrition content and chemical makeup of irradiated foods shows no impact at approved doses. The Government Accountability Office summed it up for Congress in 2010: "The safety of irradiated foods has been extensively studied and has been endorsed by the World Health Organization, CDC, USDA, and FDA," with approval in fifty-six countries.[44]

One reason consumers still shy away is that irradiation is a rare area where labeling has stuck. The FDA and USDA both require treated foods to carry a "radura" symbol indicating they have undergone the process, with the words *irradiation* or *radiation* included in the description. Though most consumers are happy to "nuke" their frozen chicken in a microwave before putting it on the grill, they don't want to see that it's been "prenuked" by their supplier. Consumer groups have also been successful in fighting adoption of the irradiation process by raising questions about added costs and by charging that irradiation would become a last-second band-aid for dirty suppliers unwilling to do the hard work of cleaning up slaughter lines and packaging centers.

"It hits people at a gut level," said Lovera of Food and Water Watch. "What is wrong with the food that you have to treat it at this level to make it safe?"[45]

It is true that cost has been a hindrance, with major suppliers fighting to shave pennies off bags of lettuce or dimes off pounds of meat in order to win the rights to shelf space at tough negotiators such as Costco, Kroger, Walmart, and more. Meat processing is more centralized in the United States and could likely withstand the added expense of mass irradiation machinery. But highly perishable produce would need to be transported long distances to warehouses large enough to make the volume-cost equation work, and farmers won't push for that without a sense the consumer would buy the result.

A failure in marketing has undercut the technology as well. Companies have tried to sneak through irradiated foods without fanfare, with a few minor exceptions, rather than touting the extra safety step as a desirable feature. Seattle food safety attorney Bill Marler points out in speech after speech to industry officials that yes, consumers appear to have an instinctive dislike for the word *radiation*.[46] But, he adds, they also have a visceral hatred for words like *E. coli* and *kidney failure* and *outbreaks*. In the worst spinach outbreaks, entire stores empty of the bagged greens, and sales don't just decline, they drop to zero. Why wouldn't more food marketers take a chance on the power of modern mass marketing to improve the reputation of a proven food safety step?

The FDA has quietly considered helping out by pondering a change of the label to less frightening words, such as *cold pasteurization*, which, while an obvious euphemistic ploy, is at least as accurate as *irradiation*. But consumer groups have risen up in arms when they hear of the proposed changes, and with an apparently disinterested food supply chain, irradiation has languished as an academic favorite and populist reject. One of the few American name brands going full force with irradiated food is Omaha Steaks.[47] All the ground beef the storied company sends out has been treated first with in-house irradiation. Sales that began from one custom butcher shop have increased every year, beyond $460 million in annual sales. "Our research and development and quality assurance teams did extensive testing to determine that irradiation had absolutely no impact on the taste or the nutritional integrity of our ground beef," said communications director Beth Weiss. After some initial questions from concerned customers when Omaha Steaks in 2000 said all of its ground beef products would be irradiated, many customers now seek out the products precisely because of the reassurance, Weiss said. The company believes it is the only one shipping treated ground beef nationwide. Though its own system is designed solely for ground beef and burgers, company officials feel irradiation would work successfully on a wide variety of consumer foods.

NANOTECHNOLOGY

The food technology of the future that may well define "eating dangerously" for years to come, nanotechnology, may already be in your refrigerator. In fact, it may actually *be* your refrigerator.

Racing far ahead of government study or control, nanotechnology—or the science of extremely small particles of known materials, with valuable properties—is already embedded in refrigerator produce drawers,[48] sippy cups, tennis jerseys, and sports socks as a bacteria-fighting agent. Packaging companies join with food giants to research unique plastic film or trays whose nanoparticles sense the growth of pathogens or spoilage and change color to warn suppliers and consumers. (Green steak package = good. Red steak package = eat vegetarian tonight.)[49]

A nanometer is one billionth of a meter. Nanotechnology manipulates basic materials like silver on a microscopic level, smaller than individual human cells. As one science blog explained it, if a nanoparticle was as big as a football, then a doughnut would be the size of New Zealand. The scent of salt on an ocean breeze is the result of natural nanoparticles permeating the mist we walk through. A Georgia Institute of Technology professor described the advance in manipulation this way: Compared to the particle control allowed by nanotechnology, existing manufacturing and chemical-mixing techniques are the equivalent of assembling LEGO blocks while wearing boxing gloves.[50] Imagine a scientist at the control of a computer screen, in touch with a silver particle thousands of times smaller than the diameter of a human hair, sending signals to the nano-messenger to maneuver in your bloodstream and destroy a concentration of *E. coli* infection in your intestines. Or imagine a golden French fry still dripping in canola oil; instead of worrying about the fats in the canola oil, you could be reading a label on the bottle of oil reassuring you that nanoparticles embedded in the oil will block cholesterol from entering your blood stream and clogging your arteries. Other researchers are look-ing for nanoparticles that could seek out the *Campylobacter* that, as we've seen, contaminates so much fresh chicken sold in the United States, and latch onto it in a way that neutralizes it as a pathogen.

The allure is that it's a wild and wide-open technology, ripe for explora-tion and exploitation. And the danger is exactly the same. You think the governments had a hard time keeping up with genetic engineering in seeds? Nanotechnology has entered American kitchens almost without government comment.

"A research strategy for addressing possible human health or environ-mental risks is not in place," ran one bleak assessment from the Woodrow Wilson International Center for Scholars Project on Emerging Nanotech-nologies. "There is no evidence that government oversight bodies are ready to conduct the kind of thorough reviews that these exciting but untested innovations demand."

Environmental and health groups warn that what we don't know about the effects of nanotechnology is as massive as the particles are small. They worry about the embedded silver particles in packaging rubbing or washing off into food. They fear for worker safety in nanoparticle manufacturing, in the way we should have worried about asbestos workers long before we actually did.[51] They wonder what happens to carbon, silver, and any number of other useful materials when they slough off products into watersheds or gather in landfills in unforeseen concentrations. The nanoparticles are powerful because the minute-sized materials behave differently in nature than larger particles of the same material. Size matters. But can that different behavior be perfectly controlled and affect only the one thing scientists want it to affect? Let's say that canola oil successfully delivers the microscopic package of cholesterol blockers into the heart. What else is it going to do once it gets there? History is an ever-growing stack of technological advances, each with a flip side of unintended consequences.

9

SO NOW YOU'RE SICK

There is no such thing as stomach flu.

It's next to impossible to do the right thing about your foodborne illness if you can't even call it by the right name. So let's dispel one of the great lingering mythologies of medicine, uttered perhaps thousands of times a day across the United States. It's not a touch of the "stomach flu" that ruins both ends, so to speak, of an otherwise normal day.

A case of the real influenza can certainly upset your stomach. And a bout with food poisoning can certainly leave parts of your body aching as if you'd been laid up with the flu. But a basket of disparate symptoms does not add up to an illness called the stomach flu.

What people call the stomach flu, for lack of a better term, is more than likely a foodborne pathogen from the list of common food-related illnesses compiled annually by the CDC. Norovirus can cause severe vomiting and diarrhea a few hours after ingestion or inhalation. *Salmonella* can cause fever and diarrhea a couple of days after eating undercooked, contaminated chicken. The parasite *Giardia* can cause an acute and then lingering gut attack a week after drinking tainted ice cubes at a foreign cafe, or drinking untreated water from a mountain stream.

There are clear medical clues, though, and some new developments in health care and food science, that can distinguish your illness from that morass of "stomach flu" suffered by millions of unknowing Americans every year. Counting backward to the camping trip where you drank untreated water can help pinpoint *Giardia* and find you the right drug to prevent weeks of ignorant suffering. Helping a doctor diagnose *E. coli* O157 can prevent lifelong kidney damage in a loved one and steer authorities toward compiling information for a widespread food recall. Making the connection between your child's vomiting and a bigger outbreak at the daycare center can contribute to the momentum building for a norovirus vaccine, one of the coming advances in pathogen control.

If a pathogen has ridden along on food and disrupted your family's life, use the following guide to narrow down the possibilities and help speed recovery. Obviously no layman's summary can substitute for sound medical advice, and only a family doctor should prescribe treatment when an illness becomes severe. But at the very least, you can be prepared, and learn how to ask the right questions.[1]

NOROVIRUS

The malady most commonly misidentified as "stomach flu" actually stems from norovirus, and it has a more accurate nickname. Imagine it stitched in red across a blue supervillain costume: PP, for "perfect pathogen."

Norovirus is omnipresent, hardy, opportunistic, adaptable, and self-preserving. Not to mention the most ominous trait—"aerosolized," which should bring to mind a cloud of millions of threatening droplets settling on surfaces passed by oblivious citizens every day. The symptoms accompanying "noro" are often characterized as "explosive," which along with "aerosolized" may fill in more of the picture than you really wanted to know.

Norovirus is by far the most common foodborne illness in the United States, though it also spreads by other viral contact methods: your airplane seat mate sneezing on your drink and your book, or a hundred people touching the same cruise ship doorknob originally grabbed by an ill partier. Its many nicknames include the "nursing home" virus, or the "cruise ship" virus, because it causes so many of the large and fast-spreading outbreaks where masses of people congregate in a small space, served by people who come into contact with a high percentage of guests.

One of the world's leading experts on norovirus wrote a paper that included a chilling tale of one outbreak investigation, which helped researchers reinforce their knowledge of the pathogen's "aerosolized" traits. A group of girls was on a road trip on a sports bus, headed to another city to play a big game. One of the athletes came down with norovirus somewhere along the way and retreated to a bathroom at a tour stop. All of us who have ever had that kind of sudden-onset stomach bug can imagine the private horror show of that bathroom: the back-wrenching nausea, the mad dashes back to the toilet stall, the gasping pauses at the sink for a splash of cold water on the back of the neck. Someone on the team had brought into that bathroom a plastic shopping bag filled with food for the team lunch, and that unfortunate cloud of illness settled all over the bathroom, including onto the bag. The sick girl left the athletic tour, but that food bag stayed with the team. The sick girl never touched it. But when the other team members ate their lunch, they were touching the bag that had sat in the middle of the pathogen cloud, then opening food, then putting hand to mouth and passing germs around the team.

Seven of the eleven girls who handled the shopping bag or its food contents also got sick with norovirus. When a norovirus sufferer walks through a public area, they leave an invisible stain across a mind-boggling number of surfaces, much like *Peanuts'* Pigpen. In researching other outbreaks, scientists have found norovirus lurking in light fixtures, among other "that's not possible!" locations. In another notorious outbreak, 2,700 people got sick from one strain—traceback researchers found all of them were connected to forty-six different weddings. The forty-six weddings all used the same bakery for the cake, and a baker's illness there was where it all began.

Elsewhere, illness tracers found 115 norovirus victims who had all eaten sandwiches made by one sub shop employee.

Norovirus causes twenty-one million U.S. cases of gastroenteritis a year, with more than five million of those delivered on or in food. The food cases alone in the United States cause about fifteen thousand hospitalizations, and 150 deaths. Worldwide, the virus may cause about two hundred thousand child deaths a year, especially in nations without the medical facilities to treat the debilitating, acute diarrhea and dehydration that can define an unattended case. (Some literature still occasionally refers to it as "Norwalk," after an Ohio city with a major outbreak of the illness in the 1960s.)

What makes norovirus so perfect in such an awful way? CDC researcher Aron Hall, a veterinarian who is one of the world leaders on the virus, listed the reasons. It's highly contagious, and in an epidemiologist's phrase, "well-shed." Imagine that cloud coming off Pigpen: one gram of feces, for example—the weight of a paper clip or dollar bill—can contain five million doses of norovirus. It can survive two weeks on a surface by being resistant to both heat and cold, and in a stable, refrigerated environment, it can survive for months. Norovirus is also clever enough to make many people sick without making many of them too sick; in other words, it does not kill its host. Those people recover, and because norovirus is constantly evolving, they do not build up full immunity to the next slightly different strain of the same virus. They are ready to play host again, and norovirus is happy to be a return guest.

Though most people who get norovirus are only symptomatically sick for one to three days, they are shedding the virus for weeks in their stool, mostly without knowing it. They may think their family is in the clear a week after their illness, but if the recovered family member serves food and doesn't practice careful hygiene, that norovirus cloud is ready and waiting.

The high survivability and voluminous "shedding" inherent to norovirus are two of the factors that landed it the dubious status of the Cruise Ship Virus. Even more accurate would be the Nursing Home Virus—by far the largest number of identified outbreaks of norovirus take place in nursing homes, where residents may have a hard time maintaining hygiene and where aides circulate from room to room many times a day, touching beds, hand rails, bathroom fixtures, doorknobs, and TV remote controls.

The virus can be a nightmare in the restaurant business as well, since it can be added into food at any stage of preparation and service while surviving almost every step of the way.

Detecting the outbreaks of norovirus is a greater challenge because the retail medical community isn't yet set up to look for the superbug. The average doctor's office or lab does not have a norovirus test kit, allowing clusters of cases to develop and multiply long before a public health agency can make all the connections.

Many foodborne illnesses share symptoms, but there are a few ways to zero in on what you or a family member might have. The incubation period for norovirus illnesses averages about twenty-four hours after contact, which is longer than a food illness caused by a toxin and shorter than the waiting period for *Salmonella* or *E. coli* to manifest.

Norovirus causes diarrhea, as in other gastrointestinal illnesses, and it is often quick onset—severely, if temporarily, debilitating. (How do we define debilitating? Curled up on a bed or a bathroom floor while calling for your mommy, and not being able to venture more than a few feet from a bathroom while the intestines are churning.) But one key to norovirus is the addition of vomiting, which can be frequent and severe, to accompany the diarrhea. The virus inflames both the stomach and the intestines. The terrible feeling for a few hours at both ends, soon followed by what can be wrenching body cramps and soreness from all the upheaval, are signs of norovirus whipping through to make your part of the universe miserable. You may also have a low-grade fever.

Generally healthy people, in the wide range between childhood and late senior years, need not worry too much about norovirus. It's awful while it's happening, yes, and will make many people beg for relief in the middle of the night, but the symptoms are usually dangerous only to the ego. Issues to look out for include severe headaches, light-headedness, and crippling fatigue that could signal dangerous dehydration. Children, the elderly, and pregnant women need to be watched more closely, since the fever and dehydration could exacerbate other medical issues.

The treatment for norovirus is time. Rest, sleep, distract yourself with favorites in your movie queue, and let the microbial invaders flush out of your body. Start sucking on ice chips when you think you might be able to hold something down, and progress to small sips of water if that goes well. Don't worry about eating any time soon; the best trick is to replace lost fluids as soon as you can tolerate them.

For those suffering an acute case that feels more dangerous, a visit to the doctor or emergency room might result in a prescription for an antinausea drug or an IV drip to more quickly replace fluid when the stomach still can't hold any. When the prospect of swallowing something other than water finally feels tolerable, some acetaminophen will help with a lingering headache or other body throbs left behind by heaving episodes.

Because norovirus sheds in such enormous quantities even after most symptoms are gone, public health officials ask parents to keep their children home from school for three days after the diarrhea has resolved in order to protect other children in close-contact settings. Scrub down the bathrooms, doorknobs, counters, and other high-contact areas with bleach-based disinfectant to stop noro from taking down anyone else in the family.

SALMONELLA

A case of salmonellosis caused by the *Salmonella* bacteria may be hard to distinguish at first from norovirus or other pathogens. But there are a few telling clues, and *Salmonella* also comes with some added dangers that make sorting out those clues a worthy venture.

Salmonella bacteria is almost always delivered to humans by the foods they eat. A significant number of cases, though, are caused by contact with pets and other animals, particularly turtles and reptiles. Moms who yell at their kids to put the turtle down and wash their hands are far from crazy—thousands of cases a year result from kids handling pets and then going straight to snack time.

The foods that turn up most often in tracebacks are undercooked poultry, raw or undercooked egg products, ground beef, and salad greens like spinach and mixed lettuce. If a meal or a snack with any of those suspect items comes to mind during the first stages of a family bout with stomach illness, note it down.

The CDC estimates about 1.4 million U.S. cases of salmonellosis a year. The average case of salmonellosis takes slightly longer to incubate than most norovirus cases. Symptoms are likely to appear eighteen to seventy-two hours after ingesting the bacteria, while many norovirus cases have shown up within twenty-four hours after contact.

The early symptoms match the usual list in any stomach-centered malady. Vomiting, headaches, fever, aches, diarrhea. One thing to watch for is diarrhea becoming bloody, which is a marker for *Salmonella*. The symptoms also can last much longer than typical norovirus, with the body feeling wracked for four to seven days in many patients.

If you need a doctor's attention and they suspect *Salmonella*, they will seek lab testing. But those results can take days, so your medical group will be treating the symptoms or even the bacteria itself before that. Dehydration is the main thing to watch for early in the illness, again especially with younger patients, the elderly, or those with previously compromised immune systems from another condition.

There are a number of different strains of this bacteria, though *Salmonella enteridis* is by far the most common.

Those patients still feeling terrible a few days into the illness will likely hear about a possible bacterial cause and ask for antibiotics to fight the salmonellosis. But they may get a fight from their doctor if they are exhibiting "normal" symptoms, however debilitating, with no complications. Overuse of antibiotics is part of what has gotten the world into more trouble with *Salmonella* in the first place. Fast-feeding livestock operations have put so much antibiotic in animal feed because preventing illness preserves profits that *Salmonella* over time developed resistant strains. As with overtreatment of childhood ear infections, the medical community wants to avoid creating superstrains and knocking more medicines from the shrinking list of effective antibiotics. And perhaps the more relevant problem: for people with those basic symptoms, antibiotics have not been shown to speed up recovery. In some research, those who were put on antibiotics had more relapses than untreated patients.

Where *Salmonella* gets worse is when it survives the stomach and intestines and moves into the bloodstream, creating a more dangerous blood infection. It can also move into other organs. This is when it becomes enteric, or typhoid, and since most Americans are not routinely immunized for typhoid, the medical problems become very serious. About 30 percent of these cases develop a telltale chest and torso rash that can help doctors identify the course of the illness.

Typhoid *Salmonella* cases present other special problems, including the possibility of long-term carriers. People can shed the bacteria and endanger those around them for years, sometimes without any idea they are putting people at risk. "Typhoid Mary" carried this version, and she infected dozens of members of various families from her position as an itinerant household cook in the early 1900s. Signs of *Salmonella* reaching the typhoid stage include fever spikes to 104 degrees or more, slow heartbeat, and inflammation in the stomach and intestines.

E. COLI

The beginnings of an *E. coli* episode may seem like a repeat of other foodborne illness descriptions, but the special dangers of certain bacteria strains make it all the more important to distinguish if you and your medical provider suspect it as a cause.

E. coli has been around, and inside, all of us for as long as we've been eating and living in an imperfectly clean world. Various strains of the bacteria are part of the human and animal intestinal system. But a few strains attacking humans from outside sources can cause bloody diarrhea, kidney failure, and in extreme cases, death. The one we've been hearing the most about in recent years is *Escherichia coli* O157:H7, which has been responsible for many of the hamburger- and spinach-related outbreaks that brought food safety awareness in the United States to new levels.

E. coli symptoms can arrive quickly, but their incubation window stretches wider than some of the other pathogens, up to eight days in some cases, compared to a day for many norovirus cases or one to three days for *Salmonella*. Once it appears, though, it is much more associated with severe diarrhea, and eventually bloody diarrhea, than with the double-whammy of vomiting from other pathogens. Severe abdominal cramps are a common accompaniment to the frequent diarrhea.

Doctors will likely ask about foods eaten, but the long incubation period for *E. coli* can make that discussion a challenge. Undercooked hamburger is highly suspect, since ground-up cattle parts bring all the potential pathogens clinging to the surface of meat deep into the heart of the food, where cooking temperatures take longer to penetrate. Other outbreaks have eventually been traced back to improperly washed spinach and other salad greens, or alfalfa sprouts that food safety officials constantly find problematic.

Dehydration from the loss of body fluids, as we've said with the other illnesses, is a prime danger from *E. coli*, particularly with children, who have less margin for fluctuation. So keep a careful eye on that; doctors will recommend replacement fluids and even resort to an IV if there's no other way to deliver the vital replenishment.

Not all labs test automatically for *E. coli*, but the doctor should seek that form of test, especially if bloody diarrhea is present. In the meantime, the other signs to be watchful for are markedly white pallor that could indicate the beginnings of anemia, and failure to produce urine. A halt to urine could be a sign that *E. coli* has begun breaking down kidney tissues, which are a prime target for the bacteria. That can lead to hemolytic uremic syndrome, or HUS, which develops in about 10 percent of children under age ten who have an *E. coli* infection. The syndrome usually shows up, if it does at all, about a week after severe diarrhea has begun. For some patients, dialysis can prevent organ failure; more severe cases can lead to permanent kidney loss and the need for lifetime dialysis or transplant.

Antibiotics are not usually recommended to fight *E. coli*'s foodborne illness symptoms, and treatment focuses on helping the body get over the symptoms, whether by adding fluids or through more drastic measures such as the blood cleansing provided by dialysis.

All *E. coli* O157 cases should be reported to local health authorities to help them isolate and recall contaminated foods that could still be on the market. Shared reporting can also alert local medical offices to catch other undiagnosed patients early enough in their illness to make a difference.

HEPATITIS A

Hepatitis A is an oddball among the common foodborne illnesses, because it is easily—if not cheaply—prevented. There is a highly effective vaccine for this less debilitating strain of hepatitis, proven safe and affording twenty years of immunity. But because it can cost $40 or more, and since nearly everyone who gets Hepatitis A recovers without lingering effects, it is usually recommended only for people traveling to less-sanitary countries, or for those who work in food service and other sensitive roles. Public health officials hesitate to add new mandatory vaccines to the growing list of citizenship requirements, and few players in America's bloated health care budgets are volunteering to pick up the cost.

Hepatitis A is commonly passed between carriers and the foods they handle after failing to properly wash their hands. The virus inflames the liver and takes ten to fifty days to incubate, challenging efforts to pin down any foods responsible through a normal traceback operation. Frequent symptoms are fatigue, jaundice or yellowed skin and eyes, abdominal pain, loss of appetite, darkened urine, vomiting, fever, and periodic diarrhea. A medical guide for families from the Philadelphia Children's Hospital estimates 40 percent of city dwellers in the United States have had the virus, many without ever knowing it. Younger people are often asymptomatic, so a family may not recognize they have a problem until a parent of the virus-carrying child also gets sick and receives a test.

The illness can last about two months before resolving, though some symptoms may linger on for some patients. Once it resolves, it does not recur, and the body is eventually rewarded for fighting off the virus with the benefit of lifelong immunity. There are no specific treatments for those with a normal case of Hepatitis A, though to protect the compromised liver, patients are told not to drink alcohol and to cut down on fatty foods.

For those considering the vaccine, remember it takes two weeks afterward to gain full protection. Patients getting over a case should talk to their doctor about protecting others if they have children at home or work in daycare or food service. They may be told to stay away from food contact or take extra precautions for some time.

CAMPYLOBACTER

Campylobacter is a parallel bacteria to *Salmonella* in many ways, sharing symptoms and some common methods of transmission. Like *Salmonella*, it likes to ride along in packages of raw chicken and eggs, but it is also common in shellfish and other seafood, and in pigs, goats, and sheep. Not all medical professionals are in the practice of looking for it specifically, even if they suspect a foodborne illness, so it has been one of the more difficult pathogens for public health officials to estimate.

The incubation period for the most common form, *Campylobacter jejuni*, is one to seven days, and the illness starts with fever, headache, muscle aches, and abdominal pain. It can progress to vomiting and frequent bloody diarrhea, with as many as ten bowel movements a day. The most severe symptoms are likely to be over in less than a week, though minor symptoms may reappear for weeks. Antibiotics for the treatment of *Campylobacter* are debated in the medical community, as it is similar to many pathogens that usually run their course without permanent damage in healthier patients. Antibiotics can slow the natural progression of the illness without greatly altering symptoms. Many doctors also recommend against antidiarrheal drugstore remedies: better to let the bacteria pass through the system. A small number of cases can lead to the more serious Guillain-Barré syndrome, a neurological disorder creating nerve tissue damage. Dehydration or diarrhea lasting more than five days usually prompts the testing for a foodborne illness, and more medical attention.

SHIGELLA

Shigella targets young children and is one of the major causes of dysentery, or bloody diarrhea, in the United States and around the world. Public health officials suspect hundreds of thousands of cases nationally each year, many of them not formally detected.

Children twelve months to four years are vulnerable because of the habits of the young: touching everything, including less clean parts of themselves, putting those same fingers or toys in the mouth, and hugging or tumbling with other children. Daycare centers are hotspots for *Shigella*, as with rotovirus, before the latter was successfully targeted by a popular vaccine. Aiding and abetting the insidiousness of *Shigella* is the tiny amount needed for an infection, with only a few cells required for transmittal. Pediatricians in Philadelphia warned in their *Shigella* guide that toilet paper is not a thick enough barrier to stop transmission, making thorough hand-washing all the more essential in kid-care settings. People can be carrying infectious levels in their intestines without getting sick themselves, distributing the potential mystery without knowing it.

"*Shigella* is so infectious that you could catch it from an infected person who loaned you his pen just long enough for you to sign your name," according to the Philadelphia manual. *Shigella* can also be picked up while swimming in dirty water, as with *E. coli*.

The incubation period with *Shigella* is two to four days, but it has been known to be shorter or longer. Symptoms range from a barely remarked upon case of diarrhea to frequent bloody or mucus-laden diarrhea, along with fever and severe cramps. Most providers will test for a range of pathogens once diarrhea becomes bloody, but it can take five days for *Shigella* to grow in the testing lab. *Shigella* is one of the few pathogens for which doctors agree on antibiotics and prescribe them, in part because they can help stop the shedding of the bacteria to others. You should ask your doctor, though, about local instances of antibiotic resistance and how the prescribed medicine for *Shigella* matches up with those trends. The antibiotics should make a difference in two to three days. In rare cases, *Shigella* produces a toxin that causes seizures; in other rare cases, it can settle into joints and cause lifetime arthritis issues.

Even without treatment, the illness should last no longer than two to seven days. *Shigella* wins nastiness points by failing to provide lifetime immunity after a case; yes, you can get it more than once. Some medical advisors will push for the whole family of a *Shigella* victim to get tested in order to slow the spreading of the easily communicated disease.

LISTERIA

Listeria is a smaller but deadlier entry in the list of foodborne pathogens.

The bacteria is common in the environment, and it spreads to food by anything from dirty factory equipment to birds leaving droppings across a farm field. *Listeria monocytogenes* from just one packing shed at one farm was the culprit in the 2011 outbreak involving Colorado cantaloupe, killing at least thirty-three people and eventually becoming the worst food-illness disaster in modern U.S. recordkeeping. It can cling to the netted rind of cantaloupe, or hide between slices of deli ham; perhaps most insidious of all, it loves cool weather and will multiply rather than retreat in the refrigerator, just where consumers think they are safely storing their food.

Listeriosis kills one in four people who get the illness because it attacks at the ends of the spectrum: elderly people with wilting immune systems or who may be fighting off cancer or other problems, and young pregnant women and their babies, whose immune systems partially shut down in order to avoid rejecting the growing fetus. Miscarriage and deaths of recent newborns are two of the sadder consequences of *Listeria*. A long incubation period also complicates identification and treatment—listeriosis can appear as long as seventy days after eating contaminated food, with the average onset in about three weeks.

Symptoms tend to mock influenza at the beginning, making it a challenge for unsuspecting doctors to diagnose in isolated occurrences. Fever, chills, sore throat, headache, and muscle ache lead off the reaction. Elderly patients can descend into meningitis and sepsis. Like other healthy adults, pregnant women may have ingested *Listeria* without knowing it and without developing the illness, while still passing it on to their vulnerable, developing baby. Tissue samples are grown in a lab to detect suspected listeriosis. Courses of antibiotics for pregnant women can help protect the baby, which is at risk of having the infection spread to vital organs. The fetus can also pick up *Listeria* in utero and then not exhibit major symptoms until some time after birth; in a newborn or infant, signs include those of meningitis, such as a bulging soft spot on the head, irritability, lethargy, and lack of appetite.

Many of the Colorado cantaloupe victims were in their eighties or beyond—just think of all the cantaloupe on the menus of nursing homes, where comfort food, nutrition, and easily chewed foods are a priority. *Listeria* could become an even more prominent preoccupation for food safety officials as the U.S. population continues to age.

CLOSTRIDIUM PERFRINGENS

Clostridium perfringens could be called the "cafeteria disease." It arises from a bacteria that exists widely in the natural and man-made environment as spores, which then take advantage of moderate temperatures to reproduce rapidly and rise to a contamination level, threatening illness to humans that ingest them. Food becomes more vulnerable to that kind of bacteria growth when it's left out to cool too slowly, or servers fail to heat it up again to a level that kills off the new bacteria. Imagine slabs of roast beef sitting on poorly tended steam tables at a convention hall, or a buffet of neglected scrambled eggs cooling and congealing at a Las Vegas hotel. *Clostridium perfringens* causes an estimated one million cases of illness in the United States each year, carried and spread from the intestines of humans and wild or domestic animals. Once ingested by humans through food, the bacteria colonize and spread, causing intense stomachaches and diarrhea, along with cramps, according to the FDA's "Big Bug Book."

Symptoms begin about eight to twenty-two hours after eating the contaminated food, so it's a relatively short incubation that can make traceback a little easier. In relatively healthy people, symptoms are usually over within twenty-four hours, although minor complications for some patients can last up to two weeks. Any deaths associated with *Clostridium* are from the ever-present gastrointestinal complication of dehydration after losing fluids. A rarer form of illness caused by *Clostridium perfringens* arises from bacteria creating necrosis in the intestines, called necrotic enteritis.

The illness can be diagnosed by its symptoms, though they, of course, overlap with many gastrointestinal problems. Fecal testing can confirm it, but many of the outbreaks go undetected because general practice doctors rarely test specifically for *Clostridium perfingens*. Tests can take one to three days to return results. Health officials who are alerted to potential cases can also go looking for food sources and get those tested for *Clostridium*; confirming the source can force institutions to throw away bad food and overhaul their serving methods.

Treatment usually consists of waiting and sympathy, accompanied by rehydration measures if there is extensive loss of fluids, particularly in children. Antibiotics are not recommended. For home cooks, the lesson from *Clostridium* is that food sitting out between 68 degrees and 140 degrees Fahrenheit is vulnerable to many kinds of bacterial growth. Cool it down quickly or heat it up sharply before serving.

TOXINS AND PARASITES

Though we will not attempt to be exhaustive in detailing every virus, bacteria, parasite, or toxin that can ride along on bad food or water, a few more are worth a mention. Most of them account for only infrequent outbreaks or affect a small number of the people targeted by foodborne pathogens.

A "staph" infection commonly associated with hospital surgery or untreated wounds can also come in the form of food poisoning, and often does. *Staphylococcus aureus* bacteria are ever-present in our environment and often arrive on food from unknowing food service workers and handlers. The bacteria produce toxins that are not cooked out of foods by heat. It is estimated to cause hundreds of thousands of cases a year, but very few are officially reported since the illness, while sometimes violent, comes in as little as thirty minutes after contact and is often gone in a day.

Giardia infection is considered a backpacker's problem, because of its strong association with drinking stream water tainted with cattle manure or other animal-feces runoff. But it's also a dog-owner's problem, and a day-care problem, and an open-water swimmer's problem. The parasite resides and grows in the intestines of many life forms, and it is one of the main reasons American backcountry users need to filter, boil, or chemically treat any local water they want to drink. Dogs can pick it up in many outdoor settings, getting the same diarrheal symptoms themselves and bringing it back home for transmission to their people. Giardiasis can range from "greasy stools that float," according to the CDC, to stomach cramps and nausea, to gaseousness and dehydration. Doctors might need more than one stool sample over multiple days to complete a test. Prescription drugs can help speed up recovery significantly, though people do recover on their own.

Toxoplasmosis is a parasite that infects millions of Americans but which rarely erupts into symptoms in those human carriers. It's most often ingested in undercooked meat, in particular pork, lamb, and venison. Cat feces are another transmitter, threatening some cat owners who are not careful about handling and hygiene. Symptoms often feel like a long-term flu, with aches and pains and swollen glands for a month or more. Occasionally patients develop a more severe case, including an ocular form of the illness that should be treated by eye doctors.

Streptococcus bacteria ingested through food can induce the same sore throat symptoms more commonly associated with an airborne or environmental contagion; other forms of foodborne strep can cause gastrointestinal problems that feel more like one of the better-known food poisons.

Some naturally occurring substances become toxins when concentrated too much in food, or in humans who eat too much of one thing. Snappers and other fish that fatten on algae near reefs can produce ciguatera poisoning, which creates a telltale numbing of the lips and tongue as a warning sign. Many diners avoid shellfish in summer months because of the various poisons they can produce after growing in hot-weather algae blooms. Forms of botulism still exist, though poisonings or outbreaks are rare compared to the size of its lingering legend as a foodborne danger. There are honey intoxications from eating too much in a season when bees used too many rhododendrons; there are molds that grow on peanuts, and city water systems that occasionally harbor a *Cryptosporidium* scare. But stick to learning the dangers of what the FDA likes to call the Big Five—norovirus, *Salmonella*, *Shigella*, Hepatitis A, and *E. coli* O157:H7—and you'll be well prepared to handle the great majority of food safety problems your family will likely ever face.

10

EATING HEALTHY AND EATING SAFE: NO, THEY AREN'T THE SAME THING

Go locavore. Eat organic. Find farm-fresh eggs from chickens that roam free to scratch the dirt and peck for bugs. Share half a butchered cow in a joint order with your neighbor, choosing it from a bucolic ranch with rolling green hills and no hormones or antibiotics mixed into the feed. Order your never-frozen Thanksgiving turkey directly from the farmer instead of shopping with the masses tossing hard-as-a-rock birds around the bin at the supermarket in search of the perfect centerpiece. Stroll through the farmers' market each week, sampling watermelon and homemade sausages and loaves of bread full of hearty seeds and grains. Go ahead—these are all wonderful ways to live. You'll develop a greater appreciation for the people who raise our food and, at the same time, help bolster the local economy.

But while you are doing all of this, don't be naïve enough to assume you are less likely than traditional grocery store shoppers to pick up a dangerous food pathogen along the way.

Eating healthy, or organically, or locally, has its benefits—fewer pesticides, more humane treatment of animals, less fossil fuel burned to transport the bananas from Chile or the hamburger from who knows where—but it has not been found to reduce the risk of foodborne illness.

Still, there are ways to seek the best in healthy, local eating and—at the same time—do your best to avoid foodborne illness. The most important thing is knowing the risks and how to minimize them.

Studies have found lower levels of chemicals in organically farmed food and hormone-free meats, but they have not determined these foods are less likely to make people sick from *Salmonella* or *E. coli* or *Listeria*. After all, organic foods are still grown or raised in and on dirt. Birds fly overhead, leaving bacteria-laced droppings behind. Wild animals trot through the farm fields. The closer to nature, the closer to bacteria, in all its good and bad forms, is usually how it goes. Again, that's why frozen chicken nuggets and boxes of crackers aren't the usual suspects behind the nation's worst outbreaks.

"Organic certification does not address food safety. Food safety is not part of the equation," said Dr. Michael Doyle, director of the Center for Food Safety at the University of Georgia. "Just because the government has this certification program, it doesn't mean it's safer."[1]

In fact, some studies have found that organic food might be slightly more likely to contain bacteria than conventionally grown or raised food. This is at least in part linked to fertilizer. In place of nitrogen-based fertilizers, organic farmers often use manure, which is teeming with bacteria, *E. coli* in particular. To make it safe, farmers are supposed to cook it first, ideally to 165 degrees. Compost it, toss it in an outdoor oven, flip it often enough to make sure the heat penetrates all the way through and cooks out the bacteria. The process can take days or even weeks. "You have a very good possibility of not getting it all, raising the risk of spreading *E. coli* on the crop," said David Lineback, senior fellow at the Joint Institute for Food Safety and Applied Nutrition at the University of Maryland. "A lot of people don't take the time."[2]

That sounds risky, perhaps, until you consider that a few decades ago, farmers simply shoveled manure straight from the stalls to the crops, unaware of the harmful bacteria it contained. But back then, people who died of foodborne illness weren't likely to figure out what was killing them, either.

These days, even though food safety officials are quite aware that manure contains potentially deadly pathogens, that doesn't mean inspectors are checking organic farming operations on a monthly or even yearly basis to make sure they are properly sanitizing their manure before they toss it on as fertilizer. "Who knows whether the manure is reaching 165 degrees, and also, all it takes is a little piece," said Jeff Nelken, a food safety expert whose company trains restaurants, grocery stores, and other retailers on how to protect against foodborne illness. "Nothing has shown that there is any less bacteria in organic."[3]

Here is another cause for concern when it comes to choosing small, organic farms: some of the nation's food safety rules apply only to farms with a certain herd size. The FDA's 2009 "egg rule," for example, applies to farms that have at least three thousand laying hens, not the little farmer with thirty hens who sells eggs at the local garden center. The rule requires testing the flock for disease, refrigeration, and safe transport, all intended to cut down on the risk of *Salmonella* bacteria. *Salmonella* infection can reside in a hen's ovaries and get transmitted to the egg, usually in the egg white.

The egg rule requires all large egg producers that don't pasteurize their eggs to adopt safety measures, which also include pest control programs—targeting rodents and flies that have access to feed troughs—and testing eggs and the chicken's environment for bacteria, refrigerating eggs at the farm and during shipping, and not sending raw eggs to stores if *Salmonella* is found in the flock.[4]

Federal authorities estimate the egg rule will save numerous lives. Yet food safety advocates say the FDA could have spared many lives and illnesses already if the agency had not stalled on passing the egg rule, and if it had given it more punch.

British egg producers have been vaccinating their hens against *Salmonella enteritidis* for more than a decade, nearly eradicating those types of human illnesses in England from eggs. In 1997, the year vaccine trials began, there were 14,771 reported cases in England and Wales of *Salmonella enteritidis* PT4, according to a report by the *New York Times*. By 2009, there were only 581 cases, a 96 percent decline, according to data from the Health Protection Agency of England and Wales.[5]

But the FDA, in passing the egg rule in 2009, did not include flock vaccinations as part of the regulation. Federal officials said there was not enough evidence that instituting a vaccination program would cut down on human illness. The vaccination would have cost less than a penny per dozen of eggs.[6]

Many large egg producers in the United States vaccinate their hens even though it is not a federal requirement. But what about the people who don't buy their eggs from a mass producer trucking them by the thousands to supermarkets across the nation? One argument on their side is that smaller, organic farmers pay more attention and take more care with their animals. Their farms and hen houses, one hopes, do not contain giant piles of animal waste that attract a larger-than-normal amount of mice and flies. They don't pump their animals full of antibiotics to prevent them from picking up the kinds of diseases that spread rapidly in overcrowded quarters. Does that mean cage-free eggs are safer?

Not necessarily, said Michele Jay-Russell, program manager and research microbiologist at the Western Center for Food Safety at the University of California.[7] "The data doesn't show that there is any difference" between eggs from the grocery store or a backyard flock, said Jay-Russell, who keeps her own hen house and supports city ordinances making it easier for city folks to raise their own laying hens. "They do need to be aware that just loving them and feeding them organic food does not prevent them from having *Salmonella*," she said. Jay-Russell recommends checking out whether an egg supplier has a clean coop with fresh food and water, whether there are signs of rodents, and whether the eggs are refrigerated after they are plucked from nests. "Whether it's a big operation or a little operation, if they don't have rodent control, they can run into problems," she said.

It's true eggs can sit at room temperature for hours and seem fine. Not so many years ago, supermarkets kept eggs at room temperature, not in the refrigerated section. But that was before scientists understood the growth patterns of *Salmonella* bacteria. "The chicken has a pretty high body temperature, even higher than humans, and the *Salmonella* likes the warm temperature," Jay-Russell said. "That's the ideal condition to grow. Refrigeration stops the growth."

The more numerous the *Salmonella* bacteria on or inside the egg, the more likely it is that bacteria will cause an infection. Eggs sometimes are contaminated with *Salmonella* on the inside, which is why it's recommended not to eat runny eggs or use raw eggs in cooking, such as in salad dressing or chocolate mousse. "There is a personal decision in all that," Jay-Russell said.

Studies comparing cage-free, organically grown eggs to those laid by caged chickens in massive facilities are contradictory. A 1994 study from California found one type of *Salmonella* was found in just 1 percent of caged hens, compared to 50 percent of free-range hens. Other European studies have found the opposite.[8]

Of all the thousands of strains of *Salmonella*, the one most commonly found in eggs is called *Salmonella enteritidis*. The strain lives in the guts of healthy animals, especially poultry and rodents, and it can be carried by flies. It can hang out in dirt and chicken, turkey, or rodent feces, and then contaminate the surface of eggs. It can spread to the rest of the flock through contaminated food, wild birds, and rodents. It can even spread from one farm to another on a worker's clothing, Jay-Russell said.

Since we're talking about eggs, it's worth knowing the difference between free-range and cage-free labels. Free-range means the chickens that laid the eggs had a bit of free time to wander outside but still could have spent much of their lives confined in barns. Cage-free means they were not confined to cages but still could have lived in close nesting quarters.

When it comes to that half-a-cow purchased from the rancher a few towns away, or the ham picked up at a nearby hog farm, treat them as if they are just as likely to contain bacteria as the beef and pork purchased at the grocery store. That means you must cook them well enough to kill any harmful pathogens. Get out the meat thermometer, again. Local meat is often butchered at a local shop, which could mean a smaller facility that might process one or two animals each day or only a handful each week. Studies show those smaller operations tend to have a slightly higher level of *E. coli* and other bacteria, said Dr. Dan Hale, a professor of agriculture science at Texas A&M University and a meat specialist.[9] "The data would show that there is a low prevalence in both locations," large or small, Hale said. "In reality, the very small facilities tend to be a little bit higher" when it comes to contamination levels. That's because larger plants have a more sophisticated pathogen eradication program, he said.

Take Cargill Meats as an example. The company is now considered one of the top innovators in food safety after a 2011 ground turkey *Salmonella* scare that at the time was the largest poultry recall in American history. Cargill recalled thirty-six million pounds of ground turkey that was potentially contaminated.[10] The company—which sells poultry, beef, and pork—ramped up its safety efforts after the recall scare.

"Food safety for Cargill food products is a top priority," company spokesman Mike Martin said in a 2013 interview.[11] "We understand that consumers expect to be able to purchase safe food. That's something we are putting in our body. Nobody wants to make anybody ill from a product that is produced and marketed under their name." But, he added, "We live in a world where these naturally occurring bacteria are ubiquitous in the environment. These are bacteria that are naturally and randomly occurring in nature. They are everywhere. They are in soil, water, animals, plants. The question is, how do you find them, rather than how does it happen. It happens naturally."

Martin points out there are more than 2,400 strains of *Salmonella* hanging around the planet, and only a handful of them are harmful to humans. The task of food producers is to track down what sometimes amounts to a small number of cells in a giant batch of ground meat or fresh greens. In the case of Cargill's enormous recall, it wasn't that all thirty-six million pounds of that ground turkey was contaminated, only that enough *Salmonella* cells were found in portions of the meat that the company had to recall entire lot numbers.

In the end, according to the CDC's final report on the outbreak, 136 people from thirty-four states were infected with the outbreak strain of *Salmonella heidelberg*. Almost forty were hospitalized. One died.[12]

Their cases were linked through DNA fingerprints after initial reports began pouring in from state health departments that people were falling ill from *Salmonella*. Interviews with ninety-four sick people revealed more than half of them recalled eating ground turkey in the seven days prior to the interviews.[13] Investigators bought ground turkey from five grocery stores and soon found the *Salmonella* Heidelberg—all originating from Cargill Meat Solutions Corporation in Springdale, Arkansas.

The particular strain of *Salmonella* was cause for concern because it is resistant to multiple antibiotics. Testing found that the strains that had made it into people's bodies because they ate the infected turkey were also resistant to some antibiotics. Fortunately, there were other available antibiotics that still worked.

A public health alert released in July 2011 warned customers to beware of fresh or frozen ground turkey and to cook it not just according to package directions, but to use a meat thermometer to make sure the meat reached 165 degrees. In August, Cargill recalled thirty-six million pounds of meat. The company says now that the outbreak, though devastating, pushed food safety efforts to a higher level.

Cargill's process of finding those pathogens before they latch on for the ride to supermarkets, and your kitchen, has ramped up considerably in the last couple of years. The company's meat, whether it's pork, beef, or turkey, has numerous "hazard analysis critical control points" along the production route. The control plan takes into account how often knives are sanitized and even how many cuts are made on a carcass. As is required by federal law, USDA inspectors are on site whenever a plant is slaughtering animals.

For ground turkey, Cargill instituted a high-pressurization technique that disrupts the growth of bacteria. Ground turkey is put into a cylinder-shaped, high-pressure vessel. The temperature is elevated, and the pressure blows up *Salmonella* cells. The high-pressure processing came about after the massive 2011 turkey recall. The company also added extra washes and more third-party safety audits, Martin said.

Neither Cargill nor federal inspectors were ever able to determine the cause of the *Salmonella* outbreak. "We never have been able to track it down exactly, other than it came from the birds," Martin said. "We're not sure how it got to the birds."

Like many meat companies, the animals used for Cargill's operations are not necessarily raised by Cargill. The company owns about 12 percent of the cattle it harvests and 25 to 30 percent of the pork. As for turkey, Cargill owns 100 percent of the birds that end up in grocery stores, but the vast majority of them are raised by ranchers on contract with the company.[14]

Cargill anticipated a setback in its reputation in August 2011 with a nationwide apology. "It is disappointing when things like this happen, given the level of effort," Martin said. "There was a pretty deep and sincere feeling of disappointment and concern and, to some degree, failure from the standpoint . . . that you never want to make someone ill from the food that you produce. It's been frustrating not to be able to do the 'CSI' work that would lead us to the source."

Cargill invested more than $1 billion in food safety in its North American operations over a decade. The company employs seven hundred people whose job, in some way or another, has to do with food safety. "It's a twenty-four-hour, seven-day-a-week, 365-day-a-year job," Martin said. "We feel that we have to have that kind of commitment to it because the potential for making people sick is something we want to continue to reduce. There is no upside for food companies to have people become ill from eating food that we produce."

The benefits of a large company such as Cargill are its relatively large budget for food safety and massive number of food safety scientists and technicians. The downsides, though, are also related to size, according to locavore enthusiasts. Unlike the family farmer down the road who sells his eggs and bacon directly to local customers, Cargill's mass-produced products take a longer path to consumption—from the farmer on contract, to the plant, to the truck, to the supermarket. That disconnect, some believe, can have a negative effect on food safety because some of the accountability for the freshness and safety of the food has been removed.

Whether connection to community makes food safer—at least until more studies are done—is more of a feel-good idea rather than a scientific fact. The connection between food safety and the locavore eating trend is minimal. "If anything, it could be a negative," said Dr. H. Russell Cross, head of the animal science department at Texas A&M University and former administrator of the USDA's FSIS under presidents George H. W. Bush and Bill Clinton.[15]

While large meat-processing plants are using high-pressure hot water or steam chambers and spraying organic acidic solutions, for example, smaller ones often use only the vitamin C sprays to help reduce bacteria on the carcass. Still, every plant—regardless of its size and unless it's operating illegally, like in someone's backyard barn operation—has a USDA inspector who is a veterinarian on site when animals are being slaughtered. For some, that means federal inspectors are there almost around the clock. For others, that means someone from the USDA stops by for a few hours each week during the killing process. Inspectors also must check on the processing operation, whether it's making sausage or grinding burger.

The USDA's food safety inspection program has more than ten thousand employees, including up to about eight thousand who are inspectors. Those eight thousand inspectors are in charge of checking on about six thousand processing plants. Contrast that with the FDA, which had 2,800 food-related staff to oversee 350,000 food makers. "If we really did the right thing, we would scrap both of those acts and write a new one that covers all food, and based on risk reduction," Cross said. The FDA inspection program is a "reactionary" one, he said. "They usually don't go get engaged until something goes wrong."

The USDA's inspection program is robust in comparison, Cross said. A meat-processing inspector must first see the animal alive, observe it get up and move. Any that look sickly are sent to a "suspect" pen for further observation. After the animals are killed, inspectors look at their organs and glands to make sure they are healthy. The meat then goes through pathogen kill process that typically involves steam, hot water pasteurization, and acidic acid or lactic acid sprays.

While A&M's Cross and Hale emphasize that the majority of meat is safe, they also push what many in food safety call the "three Cs." That's keep it cold; don't cross-contaminate raw meat with other foods in the shopping cart, refrigerator, or kitchen; and cook it well. Hale is one of the rare people who uses a meat thermometer all the time. He uses one in his burgers and in his eggs. "And I'm not a hyper-clean guy. I'm not OCD," Hale said. A particular study from Kansas State University sticks in his mind as he reaches for his meat thermometer.[16] The study found that a thermometer is the only reliable way to tell for sure that harmful bacteria has been cooked enough. Just because a hamburger is no longer pink on the inside doesn't mean it reached 165 degrees. Just because an egg is no longer runny doesn't mean the *Salmonella* in it has been killed. And just because the juices run clear when the chicken is stabbed with a fork doesn't mean it's done. Remember this, whether you are filling your basket at the farmers' market, picking up your annual half-cow, or selecting your meat at the supermarket meat counter.

"I've talked to a lot of consumers who think that if it's organic, they can almost eat it raw," Hale said. And that, clearly, is not the case.

It's also worth keeping in mind that not only should you cook organic meat or handle organic veggies the same way you do conventionally grown meat and produce, you should not assume that what you buy at the farmers' market is organic. In fact, it might not even have been grown locally or by the farmer whose stand is set up at the market to pass out slices of melon.

In 2011, strawberries purchased at farmers' markets and roadside stands in Oregon sickened fifteen people, including one who died, with *E. coli* O157:H7. It turned out the strawberries were grown by a farm in Newberg, Oregon, then sold to buyers who resold them at roadside stands and farmers' markets.[17]

Tracing the contaminated berries back to the farm was complicated. Almost all of the patients with identical strains of *E. coli* recalled eating strawberries from roadside stands or local farmers' markets, but that didn't immediately lead to the farm. Once the berries were on display at produce stands, there was nothing to tell them apart from berries from any other farm.[18] When investigators did find the farm, they also found deer tracks and droppings, which they suspected as the source of the *E. coli* contamination.

Farmers' markets are exempt from the Food Safety Modernization Act, signed into law in 2011. That's because the regulation does not apply to farms that sell less than $500,000 in food annually and sell directly to customers or restaurants within 275 miles or less from the farm.[19] Most safety experts aren't suggesting people avoid farmers' markets, just that consumers become educated about the risks. It's the responsibility of local health departments, already overburdened by restaurant inspections, to check on farmers' markets. That typically amounts to a walk-through to make sure foods sold from crepe or soup stands are heated properly. Yet many of the nation's outbreaks are caused by fresh produce, mainly leafy greens, berries, and melons—a farmers' market's main attractions.

Is organic produce healthier than conventionally grown?

Organic produce does not contain more vitamins than conventionally grown fruits and vegetables, according to a Stanford University study.[20] The study caused such a national buzz that researchers on the project were overwhelmed by interviews and soon refused to discuss it anymore. The study, which looked at four decades of research comparing organic and conventional foods, also found organic foods were not any less likely to be contaminated by dangerous bacteria, including *E. coli*. The Stanford research did find that organic foods contained less pesticide residue, however.

"When we began this project, we thought that there would likely be some findings that would support the superiority of organics over conventional food," Dr. Dena Bravata, a senior affiliate with Stanford's Center for Health Policy, told the *New York Times* after the study was completed in 2012.[21] "I think we were definitely surprised."

Another finding of note: organic chicken and pork were less likely to be contaminated by antibiotic-resistant bacteria.

A key part of the organic, locavore movement is about seeking meat and dairy products raised without antibiotics. More studies are necessary, but the concern is that antibiotics aren't healthy for the humans who eat the meat or drink the milk from animals treated with antibiotics. Besides the risk of individuals ingesting antibiotics with their glasses of milk, there is concern that the amount of antibiotics in the food chain is helping create "superbugs"—germs that have adapted to survive and are now immune to antibiotics that used to kill them. The CDC reported that "strong evidence" exists linking antibiotics in livestock to antibiotic resistance in humans. The director general of the World Health Organization said such resistance could result in "the end of modern medicine as we know it," and issues such as strep throat or an infected cut on a "child's scratched knee could once again kill."[22]

It's rarely disputed that superbugs are formidable; the ongoing debate is over how much the food supply is contributing to the problem. Plenty of safe-food advocates rail against widespread use of antibiotics in farm animals. The issue is that some food producers have for decades added low levels of antibiotics to animal feed, not because the animals are sick but to prevent infections "that tend to occur when animals are housed in crowded, unsanitary, stressful conditions," says the Natural Resources Defense Council, which along with other food safety groups filed a lawsuit against the FDA in 2011 attempting to block the use of antibiotics in animal feed. "Feeding low levels of antibiotics to cows, pigs and chickens that aren't even sick breeds super bugs—dangerous germs that are able to fight off antibiotics that spread to our communities and families."[23] The Natural Resources Defense Council places blame for superbugs directly on overuse of antibiotics in livestock, calling it a "key factor." Here is the evidence: testing of raw meat from grocery stores has revealed that about half of it contains antibiotic-resistant bacteria. Those bacteria can latch onto other surfaces in the kitchen, including knives and cutting boards, then be ingested by humans. Also, drug-resistant bacteria has been found in water near hog operations in three states and has been detected in the air downwind of hog farms, the National Resources Defense Council reports. The group's lawsuit against the FDA is ongoing. Europe has moved faster on the issue. Several countries ban antibiotics in animal feed, although veterinarians still can prescribe them for sick animals.

"For years, the FDA has avoided taking action by simply refusing to look at the evidence," said Steven Roach, public health program director for Food Animal Concerns Trust.[24]

The FDA released new guidance in 2012 that encourages ranchers to use antibiotics only when medically necessary and with veterinarian oversight. So far, compliance is voluntary, but federal officials said they haven't ruled out future regulation.

In 2012, after a federal court ordered the FDA to address the use of routine antibiotics in animal feed, Avinash Kar, a health attorney for the Natural Resources Defense Council, said: "For over thirty-five years, FDA has sat idly on the sidelines largely letting the livestock industry police itself. In that time, the overuse of antibiotics in healthy animals has skyrocketed—contributing to the rise of antibiotic-resistant bacteria that endanger human health. These drugs are intended to cure disease, not fatten pigs and chickens."[25]

The vast majority of antibacterial drugs in this country—about 70 percent—are sold for use in livestock, and most of those are used on animals that aren't sick, according to the Union of Concerned Scientists, which also sued the FDA. Despite that, others argue that blaming antibiotic consumption of livestock isn't entirely fair. Supporters of the livestock industry say hospitals, and the medical community at large, have had a much larger impact on creating superbugs than has consumption of animals that were treated with antibiotics.

Superbugs have been found in forty-two states.[26] Among the most infamous is MRSA, an antibiotic-resistant pathogen that invades hospitals and kills an estimated nineteen thousand people each year. In the spring of 2013, the CDC said it had an alarming number of new reports of so-called Carbapenem-Resistant Enterobacteriaceae or CRE, which are especially virulent and "kill up to half of patients who get bloodstream infections." The disease looks much like pneumonia. The strength of CRE, like other antibiotic-resistant germs, has much to do with overuse of antibiotics, not in animals, but in humans. Some doctors prescribe them too easily, oftentimes because their patients demand them. The overuse allows many forms of bacteria to evolve and form resistance to common antibiotics. The cycle perpetuates: hospitals have to resort to higher-level antibiotics to treat dangerous infections, the bacteria evolve again in response to the wider presence of the new antibiotic, and so on, until in some cases there are bacteria strains that don't respond to any known antibiotic. "What consequences does that antibiotic you needed have for everybody else?" asked Dr. Michelle Barron at the University of Colorado Hospital.[27] Even flushing antibiotics down the toilet has a communitywide impact in the long run, she said.

Besides never flushing antibacterial drugs down the toilet, another "for-the-good-of-the-world" action is to seek—and pay extra for—animals and animal products raised by ranchers who pledge they will not use antibiotics. Organic animal products come from animals that have not eaten antibiotics in their food. Specifically, look for USDA Certified Organic, American Grassfed Certified, and Animal Welfare Approved products.

Many farmers have abandoned the practice of giving the whole herd "just-in-case" antibiotics, not to treat illness but to prevent it. Increasingly, that is no longer seen as ethically sound. But at the same time, it's unlikely producers of America's food will stop using antibiotics altogether.

"In my mind, it would be inhumane not to treat an animal," Dr. Hale said. "The majority of consumers would agree with that statement." Producers raising "natural" animals will treat only animals that will become sick, and then sell those animals separately and not under the "natural" label, Hale said.

As for hormones in meat, scientists have found no evidence of harm to human health. "That's more of a political, societal decision of how we want to raise our meat—not a personal health decision," Jay-Russell of the University of California–Davis said. Some consumers, for example, choose to buy milk made by cows that were not given hormones often used to ramp up milk production.

One study has found that beef that was grass fed, as opposed to the standard feed lot diet of corn, was less likely to have *E. coli* contamination. Another study showed that feeding cattle grain makes their digestive tracts abnormally acidic, and over time, the *E. coli* in their guts has learned to withstand that environment. *E. coli* from grass-fed cattle are not as accustomed to the shock of the human digestive system, which is also acidic.[28] Grass-fed beef enthusiasts also argue that their animals are much less likely to have *E. coli* on their hides when they are sent to slaughter because they have not been raised in the close quarters of a feed lot, where cattle stand in dirt and manure. There are many studies contradicting the ones mentioned here, however, so it's clear that more work is needed to determine whether cattle with more room to graze are in fact safer for humans.

Another thing to consider when you buy local beef is where the animal is processed. Watch out for backyard operations not inspected by the USDA. Some consider beef unsafe, no matter how idealic the ranch or how seemingly content the free-to-graze cattle. That's because these experts fear what is lurking in the slaughterhouse. Sarah Klein, attorney at the Center for Science in the Public Interest, doesn't feed her children red meat because she is not ready to expose them to the risks of *E. coli*.[29] "Almost all cows are carrying pathogens in their guts," she said. "Once you bring it into the slaughter facility, it's exposed to all the same things as cows raised at the feed lot. Consumers are conflating the ways that food is grown or raised with safety."

Echoed egg expert Jay-Russell: "There is a lot of naïveté going on as people go back to the locavore. There is a romanticism that doesn't appreciate the risks."

A main reason people choose to eat locally grown food, and food from small farms, is that they believe those farmers are more intimately familiar with their plants and animals and have a stronger connection—and accountability—to their communities. It's true that in many cases, food grown locally is easier to trace back to the farmer.

Consider Mile High Organics, billed as the most transparent grocer that ever existed. The Colorado company that delivers organic, local, and non-genetically modified groceries to customers' doorsteps in insulated boxes can track its food almost to the exact chicken or cow. If eggs or hamburgers were to make Mile High customers ill, a traceback to the farm could take a matter of minutes, not days.

Most items—whether a peach, an egg carton, or a bottle of milk—have stickers on them identifying not just the town they came from, but the name of the farm where they were grown. Each customer's online account includes a list of every product ordered and where it originated. If a customer received something later recalled, they would get an email or phone call directly from the company, not learn on the nightly news they should throw it out. It's this connection to the customer that provides extra motivation for farmers already trying to ensure their food is safe.

Every farm is vetted by Mile High staff, which contracts with farms through Colorado and California, among other states. Different from farms that operate on a huge scale, these farms "pay attention to every detail," said Mile High founder and chief executive Michael Joseph.[30] "These people really care about what they do," Joseph said. "They are using a lot of preventative measures in their practices. We are buying a premium product, and they fetch a really good price, as opposed to more macro-produced agriculture. This is hugely reputation-based."

The company has delivered three products later recalled since it became a certified organic grocer in 2012, including one because bits of metal had potentially fallen into bread during the mixing or baking process. "We can go to people with nearly 100 percent certainty and tell them, 'You got this product delivered to your doorstep,'" Joseph said. Or, in some cases, the company can email its customers and tell them not to fear the spinach that came in their weekly order; it's not the one on the news contaminated with *E. coli*.

Right now, having hand-selected organic produce and hormone-free, locally butchered meats delivered to the doorstep is a way of life for mostly
elite eaters. It's expensive, and it attracts only those who have the combined
forces of a roomier budget and the determination to seek out higher-quality
food. Promoters, though, feel the trend can spread to more consumers and
reach an economy of scale. "I don't buy the arguments that you can't feed
the world like this. I actually think you can," Joseph said. "A growing number of people really want that type of transparency. It's really scary to worry
your food is going to kill you."

APPENDIX A

Resources to Help You Eat Less Dangerously

Numerous sites online provide up-to-date information on specific food safety events and research on food topics:

www.foodsafety.gov is a collaboration by the major government players with a hand in the issues, from the FDA to the USDA to the CDC and the National Institutes of Health. It's a consumer-friendly clearinghouse of links to practical information and advice.

www.FDA.gov is a good starting point for the latest news on food recalls, recent foodborne illness outbreaks and many other subjects.

www.USDA.gov has a little bit of everything, from recalls in meat, poultry and egg products, to consumer food handling and cooking tips to the government's arguments in favor of irradiating consumer products.

Policy-oriented views and links are at www.foodandwaterwatch.org, which takes on topics such as keeping antibiotics out of animal feed and demanding labeling for genetically modified organisms.

Pewtrusts.org oversees research and efforts to force the government to change food safety policies.

County extension agents, often linked to your state's major agricultural research university, study best practices and try to disseminate them to farmers, distributors, consumers, students and any other group that asks. Find your local network at www.csrees.usda.gov/Extension/.

Finally, for the most consumer-accessible yet hard-hitting news on detailed food safety issues, www.foodsafetynews.com has been a reliable link. It's funded in part by plaintiff's attorney Bill Marler, a national expert in food safety who litigates cases for victims and openly calls for smarter and tougher government regulation. The site's journalists consistently break news and seek alternative opinions, while tracking current outbreaks.

APPENDIX B

Food Safety Quick Tips

AT THE GROCERY STORE

Shop for Cold Items Last

- Shop for dry goods first, then hit the cooler aisles for milk, cheese, eggs, or frozen meats. The total time from the grocery store cooler to your refrigerator should never exceed four hours.
- Put your hand inside a plastic produce bag, reach for packaged meat, then pull your hand through. That way you and your cart never touch the meat package.
- Sign up for a club card with your supermarket. If there is a recall, the grocery store can notify you that you bought the contaminated item.

Dented Cans and Bruised Fruit

- Avoid buying cans with dents on the lip or the side seam because those weak spots can provide entry for bacteria that could lead to the toxin botulism.
- Experts disagree about bruised fruit. Some say bruises can harbor bacteria, so you'd better toss it; others say buy it anyway and cut well around the damaged section.

Reusable Shopping Bags

- Wash them occasionally in your washing machine. Separate bags for produce and raw meat are a must.

PREPARING THE MEAL

Produce

- Scrub melons, apples, carrots—pretty much all fruits and veggies you are going to eat raw—with a scrubber (like the kind used for potatoes). Occasionally run the scrubber through the dishwasher on the sanitary cycle.
- Don't bother using soap or a produce-cleaning spray, because there are no data showing these work better than tap water, and soap film clings. Antibacterial cutting boards are not recommended either.
- Even wash bananas if you are going to cut them in half. As with melons and other whole fruit, a knife can drag bacteria from the peel into the fruit. The bacteria continues to grow as the uneaten half sits on the counter or in the fridge.
- Wash produce right before you eat it. Otherwise, the bacteria you didn't rinse off will continue to grow.
- The water that mists lettuce at many grocery stores might make it crisper, but it doesn't clean it. Rinse it with tap water at home and let it air dry, or pat it dry. Don't wash lettuce in a sink bath, and don't wash prewashed greens that come in a bag because it only makes them more susceptible to contamination.
- Store meat on the bottom of your refrigerator, below produce that will be eaten raw, to prevent drips of bacteria on your oranges and peppers.

Meat

- Many experts discourage rinsing meat that will be cooked because bacteria get splashed around the sink and counters. If you are cooking meat to the right internal temperature, those surface bacteria will be killed.

While Cooking

DO

- Wash your hands frequently.
- Use separate cutting boards and other utensils for produce and meat. Wash and dry between uses.

- Get a good meat thermometer, and learn how to use it.
- Heat packaged deli meat to steaming before eating. Listeria lurks in the packaging facilities and isn't deterred by refrigeration.

DON'T

- Prepare food when you are sick.
- Leave food out for longer than a couple of hours. To kill bacteria, food should be kept hotter than 135 degrees or cooler than 41 degrees.
- Eat raw eggs. If a recipe calls for raw eggs, use either the pasteurized eggs in a carton or ask your grocer to special-order eggs pasteurized in the shell.
- Use the same platter for raw chicken and cooked chicken.

CLEANUP AND LEFTOVERS

- Wipe down all used surfaces, including the refrigerator, with a clean cloth and, occasionally, a sanitizer.
- Put cutting boards, sink sponges, and scrub brushes in the dishwasher, and use the "sanitize" or "antibacterial" cycle. You can also do this with lunchboxes or other utensils.
- Discard deeply rutted or damaged cutting boards with hiding places for bacteria.
- Sanitize surfaces and the sink with a mixture of one tablespoon of bleach in one gallon of water, or another store-bought disinfectant.
- Eat leftovers within three days and cut fruit within a day. Older advice that leftovers can last a week is being discarded by some state university kitchens.
- At normal temperatures, cooked food can be left on counters about four hours. In temperatures above 90 degrees, put it away within two hours.

NOTES

CHAPTER I

1. Centers for Disease Control and Prevention, "Multistate Outbreak of *Listeriosis* Linked to Whole Cantaloupes from Jensen Farms, Colorado." Last modified August 27, 2012. Accessed April 2013. http://www.cdc.gov/listeria/outbreaks/cantaloupes-jensen-farms/082712/.

2. Consumer Reports, "How Safe Is That Chicken? Most Tested Broilers Were Contaminated." Last modified January 2010. Accessed April 2013. http://www.consumerreports.org/cro/2012/05/how-safe-is-that-chicken/index.htm.

3. James Andrews, Food Safety News, "'Restaurant A' Revealed to Be Taco Bell." Last modified February 2, 2012. Accessed April 2013. http://www.foodsafetynews.com/2012/02/analysis-restaurant-a-revealed-to-be-taco-bell/; "Acute Disease Service Summary of Supplemental Questionnaire Responses Specific to Taco Bell Exposure of Oklahoma Outbreak-Associated Cases Multistate *Salmonella* Enteritidis Outbreak Investigation November 2011–January 2012," Oklahoma Department of Health Acute Disease Service. Accessed July 2013.

4. Joel L. Greene, Congressional Research Service, "Lean Finely Textured Beef: The 'Pink Slime' Controversy," April 6, 2012.

5. Centers for Disease Control and Prevention, "Estimates of Foodborne Illness in the United States." Last modified February 2013. Accessed April 2013. http://www.cdc.gov/foodborneburden/.

6. Centers for Disease Control and Prevention, "Infections from Some Foodborne Germs Increased, While Others Remained Unchanged in 2012." Last

modified April 2013. Accessed April 2013. http://www.cdc.gov/media/releases/2013/p0418-foodborne-germs.html.

7. U.S. Food and Drug Administration, Interviews, by Michael Booth. September 2011.

8. U.S. House of Representatives, Committee on Energy and Commerce, "Report on the Investigation of the Outbreak of *Listeria monocytogenes* in Cantaloupe at Jensen Farms." Last modified January 2012. Accessed November 2012.

9. Ibid.

10. Michael Booth, "Listeria Outbreak Traced to Colorado Leaves Damaged Survivors in Its Wake." *Denver Post*, December 1, 2011. http://www.denverpost.com/news/ci_19445309.

11. Lucia Graves, "Senate Passes Sweeping Food-Safety Bill." *Huffington Post*, Last modified November 30, 2010. Accessed April 2013. http://www.huffingtonpost.com/2010/11/30/senate-passes-sweeping-fo_n_789771.html.

12. Steven Grossman, "FDA Matters: The Grossman FDA Report," interview by Michael Booth, March 2013.

13. Michael Booth, "FDA Seeks Millions for Food Safety in Wake of Colorado *Listeria* Outbreak." *Denver Post*, February 13, 2012.

14. Cindy Galli, ABC News, "Budget Cuts Will Kill Safety Program That Caught *Salmonella*, *E. coli*, *Listeria* Outbreaks." Last modified July 11, 2012. Accessed April 2013.

15. Centers for Disease Control and Prevention, "Investigation Announcement: Multistate Outbreak of *Salmonella* Enteritidis Infections Linked to Restaurant Chain A." Last modified January 2012. Accessed April 2013. http://www.cdc.gov/salmonella/restaurant-enteriditis/011912/.

16. JoNel Aleccia, NBC News.com, "Taco Bell Was Behind Latest *Salmonella* Outbreak, Oklahoma Says." Last modified February 1, 2012. Accessed April 2013.

17. Michael Booth, "FDA Criticized for Food Illness Probes, Secrecy." *Denver Post*, April 13, 2012.

18. U.S. Representative Henry Waxman, statement as chairman, Committee on Energy and Commerce, "The Outbreak of Salmonella in Eggs," Subcommittee on Oversight and Investigations, September 22, 2010.

19. U.S. Food and Drug Administration, "483 Inspectional Observations on the Egg Recall." Last modified August 26, 2010. Accessed April 2013. http://www.fda.gov/Safety/Recalls/MajorProductRecalls/ucm223522.htm.

20. Mary Clare Jalonick, "Egg Company Chiefs Give Congress Few Answers." AP, printed by U-T San Diego, September 22, 2010.

21. Gardiner Harris, "Egg Producer Says His Business Grew Too Quickly." *New York Times*, September 22, 2010.

22. Jennifer Brown, "Ill Girl's Highlands Ranch Family Sues over Dough." *Denver Post*, June 24, 2009.

23. Jeannine Stein, "The Culprit in a Cookie Dough *E. coli* Outbreak Could Be Raw Flour." *Los Angeles Times*, December 9, 2011.

24. Ibid.

25. U.S. Food and Drug Administration, "Peanut Butter and Other Peanut Containing Products Recall List." Last modified October 2009. Accessed November 2012. http://www.accessdata.fda.gov/scripts/peanutbutterrecall/index.cfm.

26. Michael Booth and Jennifer Brown, "*Listeria* Outbreak Victims Go Beyond Farm to Target Grocers, Auditors." *Denver Post*, November 7, 2011. Accessed November 2012. http://www.denverpost.com/news/ci_19279433.

27. CBS News, "Peanut CEO Takes the Fifth." Last modified September 9, 2010. Accessed April 2013.

28. Julie Schmit, *USA Today*, "Peanut Boss Refuses to Testify at *Salmonella* Hearing." February 12, 2009. Accessed August 2013.

29. CBS News, "Peanut CEO Takes the Fifth."

30. Michael Booth and Jennifer Brown, "Criminal Charges Hard to Pin on Farm Where *Listeria*-Tainted Cantaloupes Originated." *Denver Post*, November 21, 2011.

31. The Associated Press, "AP Exclusive: Owner of peanut company linked to 9 salmonella deaths is back in business." September 8, 2010, as published by FoxNews.com. Accessed November 2013.

32. Sabin Russell, "Spinach *E. coli* Linked to Cattle." *SF Gate/San Francisco Chronicle*, October 13, 2006.

33. California Food Emergency Response Team, "Investigation of an *Escherichia coli* O157:H7 Outbreak Associated with Dole Pre-Packaged Spinach." Last modified March 2007. Accessed November 2012. http://cdm16254.contentdm.oclc.org/cdm/ref/collection/p178601ccp2/id/1121.

34. Herb Weisbaum, MSNBC, republished by MarlerClark, "*E. coli* Aftermath: Where Is the Accountability?" Last modified October 24, 2006. Accessed April 2013. http://www.marlerclark.com/case_news/detail/e-coli-aftermath-where-is-the-accountability.

35. Jeff Benedict, *Poisoned: The True Story of the Deadly* E. coli *Outbreak That Changed the Way Americans Eat* (Buena Vista, VA: Inspire Books, 2011).

36. Bill Marler, MarlerClark law firm, Seattle, interview by Michael Booth, December 2011; Elaine Porterfield and Adam Berliant Mcclatchy, printed in *Spokane Spokesman-Review*, "Jack in the Box Ignored Food Safety Regulations, Court Documents Say." Last modified June 17, 1995. Accessed August 2013.

37. Benedict, *Poisoned*.

CHAPTER 2

1. *Center for Food Safety and Center for Environmental Health, Plaintiffs, v. Margaret A. Hamburg, M.D., Commissioner of U.S. Food and Drug Administration, et al.*, "Complaint for Declaratory and Injunctive Relief," CV-12-4529, U.S. District Court for the Northern District of California. Last modified August 29, 2012. Accessed December 2012.

2. Michael Booth and Jennifer Brown, "Producers Seldom Hear of Food-Safety Issues from Their Private Auditors." *Denver Post*, October 30, 2011.

3. Dina ElBoghdady, "Produce-Safety Testing Program on Chopping Block." *Washington Post*, July 12, 2012. Accessed December 2012. http://www.wash ingtonpost.com/business/economy/produce-safety-testing-program-on-chopping -block/2012/07/12/gJQAHdHWgW_story.html.

4. Renee Johnson, Congressional Research Service, "The Federal Food Safety System: A Primer." Last modified January 11, 2011. Accessed December 2012.

5. Johnson, Congressional Research Service.

6. Booth and Brown, "Producers Seldom Hear of Food Safety Issues."

7. Robert Stovicek, president of PrimusLabs, interviewed by Michael Booth, October 2011.

8. Michael Booth, "Private Audit at Jensen Farms before *Listeria* Outbreak Failed to Flag Woes." *Denver Post*, October 21, 2011.

9. U.S. House of Representatives, Committee on Energy and Commerce, "Report."

10. U.S. Food and Drug Administration, "Environmental Assessment: Factors Potentially Contributing to the Contamination of Fresh Whole Cantaloupe Implicated in a Multi-State Outbreak of *Listeriosis*." Last modified October 19, 2011. Accessed December 2012. http://www.fda.gov/Food/RecallsOutbreaksEmergencies/ Outbreaks/ucm276247.htm.

11. U.S. House of Representatives, Committee on Energy and Commerce, "Report."

12. U.S. Food and Drug Administration, "Guidance for Industry: Guide to Minimize Microbial Food Safety Hazards of Melons; Draft Guidance." Last modified July 2009. Accessed December 2012. http://www.fda.gov/Food/Guidance Regulation/GuidanceDocumentsRegulatoryInformation/ProducePlantProducts/ ucm174171.htm.

13. Center for Food Safety, et al., lawsuit.

14. PrimusLabs, "Audit Certificate, Jensen Farms." Last modified July 25, 2011. Accessed October 2011.

15. Stovicek, interview.

16. D. A. Powell et al., "Audits and Inspections Are Never Enough: A Critique to Enhance Food Safety." *Food Control* 30, no. 2 (2013): 686–91.

17. Will Daniels, chief of quality and food safety, Earthbound Farm, interview by Michael Booth, January 2013.

18. California Food Emergency Response Team, "Investigation of an *Escherichia coli* O157:H7 Outbreak Associated with Dole Pre-Packaged Spinach." Last modified March 2007. Accessed November 2012.

19. Ashlee Litkey, victim of *E. coli* food poisoning, interview by Michael Booth, February 2013.

20. Ibid.

21. Daniels, interview.

22. David Gombas, vice president, food safety and technology, United Fresh Produce Trade Association, interview by Michael Booth, October 2011.

23. Cindy Galli, ABC News, "Budget Cuts Will Kill Safety Program That Caught *Salmonella*, *E. coli*, and *Listeria* Outbreaks." July 11, 2012.

24. U.S. Food and Drug Administration, "FDA Warns Consumers Not to Eat Cantaloupes from Burch Equipment LLC of North Carolina." Last modified August 2012. Accessed January 2013. http://www.fda.gov/NewsEvents/Newsroom/PressAnnouncements/ucm313743.htm.

25. FoxNews.com, "Obama Promises Thorough Review of FDA after *Salmonella* Outbreak Sickens Hundreds." Accessed August 2013. http://www.foxnews.com/politics/2009/02/02/obama-promises-thorough-review-fda-salmonella-outbreak-sickens-hundreds/.

26. Department of Health and Human Services, 2013 Budget Request, Centers for Disease Control and Prevention, 113. Accessed August 2013. www.cdc.gov/fmo/topic/Budget%20Information/appropriations_budget_form_pdf/FY2013_CDC_CJ_Final.pdf.

27. Booth and Brown, "Producers Seldom Hear of Food-Safety Issues."

28. Sandra Eskin, director, Food Safety Campaign, Pew Health Group, interview by Michael Booth, January 2013.

29. Booth, "FDA Seeks Millions."

30. U.S. Food and Drug Administration, "Transforming Food Safety, FDA FY 2013 Budget." Last modified 2012. Accessed February 2013.

31. Ibid.

32. National Association of County and City Health Officials, "More Than Half of Local Health Departments Cut Services in First Half of 2011." Last modified October 2011. Accessed January 2013. http://www.naccho.org/press/releases/100411.cfm.

33. Alfred Almanza, U.S. Department of Agriculture, "Setting the Record Straight on the Proposed Chicken Inspection Policy." Last modified April 2012. Accessed January 2013. http://www.fsis.usda.gov/News_&_Events/NR_041312_01/index.asp.

34. Gabriel Thompson, "New Rules Mean New Hardship for Poultry Workers." *The Nation*, April 25, 2012. http://www.thenation.com/article/167561/new-rules-mean-new-hardship-poultry-workers/.

35. Ibid.

36. Office of Inspector General, U.S. Department of Agriculture, "Application of FSIS Sampling Protocol for Testing Beef Trim for *E. coli* 0157:H7." Last modified May 2012. Accessed April 2013.

37. Michael Booth, "FDA Warns Colorado Cantaloupe Farms They Will Be Tested in 2013." *Denver Post*, February 25, 2013.

38. Nature.com, "Starvation Diet: A Severe Approach to Slashing US Spending Bodes Ill for the Research Enterprise." Last modified February 27, 2013. Accessed April 6, 2013.

CHAPTER 3

1. Jennifer Brown and Michael Booth. "Initial Suspicion of *Listeria* Outbreak Led to Far-Reaching Investigation." *Denver Post*, September 22, 2011. http://www.denverpost.com/breakingnews/ci_18952250.

2. Lauran Neergaard, "CDC Chief: Spending Cuts Threaten Public Health." *Associated Press*, February 22, 2013. http://bigstory.ap.org/article/cdc-chief-spending-cuts-threaten-public-health.

3. CDC, "Multistate Outbreak of *Listeriosis* Linked to Whole Cantaloupes from Jensen Farms, Colorado." Last modified August 27, 2012. http://www.cdc.gov/listeria/outbreaks/cantaloupes-jensen-farms/index.html.

4. Alicia Cronquist, epidemiologist, Colorado Department of Public Health and Environment, interview by Jennifer Brown, February 2013.

5. "A Colorado Cantaloupe Saga," Association of Public Health Laboratories. Accessed April 18, 2013. http://www.aphl.org/aboutaphl/success/listeria/pages/default.aspx.

6. Brown and Booth, "Initial Suspicion of *Listeria* Outbreak Led to Far-Reaching Investigation."

7. Laura Gieraltowski, epidemiologist, CDC, interview by Jennifer Brown, January 2013.

8. CDC, "Multistate Outbreak of *Salmonella* Bredeney Infections Linked to Peanut Butter Manufactured by Sunland, Inc. (Final Update)." Last modified November 30, 2012. http://www.cdc.gov/salmonella/bredeney-09-12/.

9. Mary Clare Jalonick, "FDA Halts Operations at Peanut Butter Plant Linked to *Salmonella* Outbreak." *Associated Press*, November 26, 2012.

10. Jeri Clausing, "Deal Reached to Reopen NM Peanut Butter Plant." *Associated Press*, December 21, 2012.

11. Oklahoma State Department of Health, s.v. "Acute Disease Service Summary of Supplemental Questionnaire Responses Specific to Taco Bell Exposure of Oklahoma Outbreak-associated Cases Multistate *Salmonella* Enteritidis Outbreak Investigation November 2011–January 2012." And James Andrews, "Analysis: 'Restaurant A'" Revealed to Be Taco Bell." *Food Safety News*, February 2, 2012.

12. CDC, "Multistate Outbreak of *Salmonella* Enteritidis Infections Linked to Restaurant Chain A." Last modified January 19, 2012. http://www.cdc.gov/salmonella/restaurant-enteriditis/011912/.

13. Lawrence Burnsed, Oklahoma Department of Health, interview by Jennifer Brown, November 2012.

14. CDC, "CDC Investigation Announcement: Multistate Outbreaks of Human *Salmonella* Hartford and *Salmonella* Baildon Infections." Last modified August 4, 2010. http://www.cdc.gov/salmonella/baildon-hartford/index.html.

15. Taco Bell, "Statement Regarding October–November 2011 Centers for Disease Control (CDC) Investigation." Last modified February 2, 2012. http://www.tacobell.com/Company/newsreleases/feb22012statement.

16. Michael Booth, "FDA Criticized for Food Illness Probes, Secrecy." *Denver Post*, April 13, 2012.

17. Booth, "FDA Criticized for Food Illness Probes, Secrecy."

CHAPTER 4

1. Pew Health Group, "Food Import Safety: Food Safety Modernization Act." Last modified October 19, 2011. Accessed April 2013. http://www.pewtrusts.org/our_work_report_detail.aspx?id=85899365446.

2. Hannah Gould et al., Centers for Disease Control and Prevention, "CDC Research Shows Outbreaks Linked to Imported Foods Increasing." Last modified March 14, 2012. Accessed April 2013. http://www.cdc.gov/media/releases/2012/p0314_foodborne.html.

3. U.S. Food and Drug Administration, "Pathway to Global Product Safety and Quality." Last modified July 7, 2011. Accessed April 2013. http://www.fda.gov/downloads/AboutFDA/CentersOffices/OfficeofGlobalRegulatoryOperationsand Policy/GlobalProductPathway/UCM262528.pdf.

4. Ibid.

5. Robert Buchanan, University of Maryland, director of the Center for Food Safety and Security Systems, interview by Michael Booth, November 2012.

6. Buchanan, interview.

7. Anna Yukhananov, "FDA Tests Threaten Brazil Orange Juice Imports." *Reuters*, Online edition, January 11, 2012.

8. Brad Racino, "Flood of Food Imported to U.S., But Only 2 Percent Inspected." *News21*, October 3, 2011. http://www.nbcnews.com/id/44701433/.

9. Stephanie Armour, John Lippert, and Michael Smith, "Food Sickens Millions as Company-Paid Checks Find It Safe." *Bloomberg Markets Magazine*, October 10, 2012.

10. Michael Doyle, University of Georgia regents professor of Food Microbiology Director, Center for Food Safety, interview by Michael Booth, November 2012.

11. Nguyen Dieu Tu Uyen and William Bi, "Asian Seafood Raised on Pig Feces Approved for U.S. Consumers." *Bloomberg Markets Magazine*, October 10, 2012.

12. Doyle, interview.

13. U.S. Food and Drug Administration, "Melamine Contamination in China." Last modified January 5, 2009. Accessed December 2013. http://www.fda.gov/NewsEvents/PublicHealthFocus/ucm179005.htm.

14. Fred Gale and Jean C. Buzby, U.S. Department of Agriculture, "Imports from China and Food Safety Issues." Last modified July 2009. Accessed December 2012. http://www.ers.usda.gov/media/156008/eib52_1_.pdf.

15. Paul Mooney, "The Story Behind China's Tainted Milk Scandal." *U.S. News & World Report*, October 9, 2008. Accessed December 2013. http://www

.usnews.com/news/world/articles/2008/10/09/the-story-behind-chinas-tainted-milk
-scandal?page=3.

16. Jim Yardley, "More Candy from China, Tainted, Is in U.S." *New York Times*,
October 1, 2008.

17. Tania Branigan, "China Executes Two for Tainted Milk Scandal." *Guardian*,
November 24, 2009. Accessed April 2013. http://www.guardian.co.uk/world/2009/
nov/24/china-executes-milk-scandal-pair.

18. FDA, "Melamine Pet Food Recall—Frequently Asked Questions." Last
modified 2009. Accessed April 2013. http://www.fda.gov/animalveterinary/safety-
health/RecallsWithdrawals/ucm129932.htm.

19. Alex Ferguson, Food Safety News, "Melamine in Chinese Powered Milk
. . . Again." Last modified January 6, 2010. Accessed April 2013. http://www.food
safetynews.com/2010/01/melamine-in-chinese-powered-milkagain/.

20. U.S. FDA, "Pathway."

21. Samantha Olson, "Chicken from China Is Approved by USDA for Import
into US." MedicalDaily.com, September 5, 2013. Accessed September 6, 2013.
http://www.medicaldaily.com/chicken-china-approved-usda-import-us-255727.

22. U.S. FDA, *FDA's International Food Safety Capacity-Building Plan*. Washington, D.C.: U.S. Department of Health and Human Services, 2013.

23. Ibid.

24. Ibid.

25. Racino, "Flood of Food Imported to U.S."

26. U.S. Food and Drug Administration, "Transforming Food Safety, FDA
FY 2013 Budget." Last modified 2012. Accessed February 2013. http://www
.fda.gov/downloads/AboutFDA/ReportsManualsForms/Reports/BudgetReports/
UCM301409.pdf.

27. Margaret Hamburg, MD, FDA commissioner, conference call with U.S.
news reporters, July 26, 2013.

28. Ibid.

29. U.S. FDA, "Pathway."

30. USDA Food Safety and Inspection Service, "FSIS Import Procedures for
Meat, Poultry and Egg Products." Accessed March 2013. http://www.fsis.usda.gov/
wps/portal/fsis/topics/food-safety-education/get-answers/food-safety-fact-sheets/
production-and-inspection/fsis-import-procedures-for-meat-poultry-and-egg
-products/fsis-import-procedures.

31. Christopher Waldrop, director of Food Policy Institute, Consumer Federation of America, interview by Michael Booth, December 2012.

32. CBC News, "XL Foods Says Problems Fixed at Plant." Last modified October 10, 2012. Accessed December 2012. http://www.prepperpodcast.com/xl-foods
-fixed-plant/#axzz2g0hpM2NF.

33. Helen Bottemiller, "Investigation: USDA Quietly Eliminated 60 Percent of
Foreign Meat Inspections." *Food Safety News*, November 1, 2012.

34. U.S. Government Accountability Office, "FDA Needs to Fully Implement Key Management Practices to Lessen Modernization Risks." Last modified March 15, 2012. Accessed December 2012. http://www.gao.gov/products/GAO-12-346.

35. U.S. Food and Drug Administration, "PREDICT Fact Sheet." Last modified July 2012. Accessed December 2012.

36. CDC, "Multistate Outbreak of Hepatitis A Virus Infections Linked to Pomegranate Seeds from Turkey." Last modified August 3, 2013. Accessed August 2013. http://www.cdc.gov/hepatitis/outbreaks/2013/a1b-03-31/index.html.

37. Centers for Disease Control and Prevention, "*Salmonella* Montevideo Infections Associated with Salami Products Made with Contaminated Imported Black and Red Pepper, U.S., July 2009–April 2010." Last modified December 2010. Accessed December 2013. www.cdc.gov/mmwr/preview/mmwrhtml/mm5950a3.htm.

38. Dschabner, ABC News, "Big Salami Recall Related to *Salmonella* Outbreak." Last modified January 2010. Accessed December 2012. www.abcnews.go.com/blogs/headlines/2010/01/big-salami-recall.

39. Doyle, interview.

CHAPTER 5

1. Jeff Almer, son of PCA peanut butter victim, Shirley Almer, interview by Jennifer Brown, December 2012.

2. U.S. District Court for the Middle District of Georgia, *U.S. v. Stewart Parnell et al.* Accessed April 19, 2013. http://www.justice.gov/iso/opa/resources/61201322111426350488.pdf.

3. Gardiner Harris, "Peanut Products Sent Out before Tests." *New York Times*, February 11, 2009. http://travel.nytimes.com/2009/02/12/health/policy/12peanut.html?_r=0.

4. Bill Meyer, "Peanut Corp. of America Owner Stewart Parnell Refuses to Testify to Congress about *Salmonella*." *Plain Dealer*, February 11, 2009.

5. Department of Justice, Office of Public Affairs, "Former Officials and Broker of Peanut Corporation of America Indicted Related to Salmonella-Tainted Peanut Products." Last modified February 21, 2013. http://www.justice.gov/opa/pr/2013/February/13-civ-220.html.

6. Sabrina Tavernise, "Charges Filed in Peanut Salmonella Case." *New York Times*, February 21, 2013.

7. Nick Miroff and Lyndsey Layton, "Peanut Company Files for Bankruptcy Protection." *Washington Post*, February 14, 2009. http://articles.washingtonpost.com/2009-02-14/news/36869545_1_pca-peanut-products-stewart-parnell.

8. CDC, "Investigation Update: Outbreak of *Salmonella* Typhimurium Infections, 2008–2009." Last modified May 11, 2010. http://www.cdc.gov/salmonella/typhimurium/update.html.

9. Justin Prochnow, attorney, interview by Jennifer Brown, December 2012.

10. Michael Booth and Jennifer Brown, "Criminal Charges Hard to Pin on Farm Where *Listeria*-Tainted Cantaloupes Originated." *Denver Post*, November 21, 2011.

11. CNN, "Juice Maker Agrees to Pay Record $1.5M Fine over 1996 *E. coli* Outbreak." July 23, 1998. http://money.cnn.com/1998/07/23/companies/odwalla/.

12. George Raine, "Odwalla Juice Suspect before Death." *San Francisco Examiner*, April 8, 1998.

13. Leonard Buder, "Jail Terms for 2 in Beech-Nut Case." *New York Times*, June 17, 1988. http://www.nytimes.com/1988/06/17/business/jail-terms-for-2-in -beech-nut-case.html.

14. Committee on Energy and Commerce, "Chairmen Request More Details on *Salmonella* Contamination at Wright County Egg." Last modified September 14, 2010. Accessed April 20, 2013. http://democrats.energycommerce.house.gov/ index.php?q=news/chairmen-request-more-details-on-salmonella-contamination- at-wright-county-egg.

15. Ryan J. Foley, "Ex-Iowa Egg Farm Manager Pleads Guilty to Bribery." *Associated Press*, September 12, 2012.

16. Ryan J. Foley, "After *Salmonella* Outbreak, Egg Mogul Will Quit His Farms." *Associated Press*, November 22, 2011.

17. Fred Pritzker, food safety attorney, interview by Jennifer Brown, November 2012.

18. Michael Booth and Jennifer Brown, "*Listeria* Outbreak Victims Go Beyond Farm to Target Grocers, Auditors." *Denver Post*, November 7, 2011.

CHAPTER 6

1. The information in chapter 6 is a compilation of research and advice from a variety of sources, often converging, but occasionally differing in nuance or calling for more study. When opinions veer or are stated more strongly than others, we have identified sources within the text. Otherwise, a bibliography of the interviews and resources consulted includes the following: Author interviews with Marisa Bunning, assistant professor and food safety extension specialist, Colorado State University; Therese Pilonetti, manager, grocery store inspection unit, Colorado Department of Public Health and Environment; Jean Halloran, director of food policy initiatives for the advocacy arm of *Consumer Reports*; Alicia Cronquist, epidemiologist, Colorado Department of Public Health and Environment; Larry Goodridge, assistant professor of microbiology, Colorado State University; Elliot Ryser, professor of food science and human nutrition, Michigan State University; Lydia Medeiros, professor of human nutrition, Ohio State University; Douglas Powell, professor of diagnostic medicine and pathobiology, Kansas State University; Trevor Suslow, extension research specialist, plant pathology, University of

California-Davis; Dave Gombas, senior vice president of food safety, United Fresh Produce; Amanda Hitt, director Food Integrity Campaign, Government Accountability Project; Caroline Smith De Waal, director of the Center for Food Safety, Center for Science in the Public Interest; Sandy McCurdy, professor, School of Family and Consumer Sciences, University of Idaho; Michael Bartolo, extension scientist, Colorado State University; food safety officials at Costco, Whole Foods, Walmart, and King Soopers; Hugh Maguire, chief epidemiologist, Colorado Department of Public Health and Environment; Sarah Klein, senior staff attorney for food safety, Center for Science and the Public Interest; Dr. Michelle Barron, head of infectious disease control, University of Colorado Hospital; Aron Hall, DVM, Centers for Disease Control and Prevention; Sandra Eskin, director, Food Safety Campaign, Pew Charitable Trusts; Alan Lewis, director of special projects and organic compliance, Natural Grocers by Vitamin Cottage; Christopher Waldrop, director, Food Policy Institute of the Consumer Federation of America; and Steve Wilson, American Society for Quality.

Articles consulted include: Jennifer Brown and Michael Booth, "Food-Safety Experts Rethink Advice after Deadly Cantaloupe *Listeria* Outbreak," *Denver Post*, November 14, 2011; food safety guides accessible online from the U.S. Department of Agriculture, Food Safety and Inspection Service; Food and Drug Administration; the Centers for Disease Control and Prevention; and the NSF International Household Germ Study, 2013.

CHAPTER 7

1. Sarah Klein, attorney, Center for Science in the Public Interest, interview by Jennifer Brown, January 2013.

2. CDC, "Multistate Outbreak of Shiga Toxin-Producing *Escherichia coli* O26 Infections Linked to Raw Clover Sprouts at Jimmy John's Restaurants." Last modified April 3, 2012. Accessed January 2013. http://www.cdc.gov/ecoli/2012/o26-02 -12/index.html.

3. Dan Flynn, *Food Safety News*, "Jimmy John's Permanently Dropping Sprouts from Menus." February 20, 2012. Accessed January 2013. http://www.foodsafety news.com/2012/02/jimmy-johns-gourmet-sandwich-franchise/.

4. FDA, "Sprouters Northwest, Inc. Recalls Clover Sprouts and Clover Sprout Mixes because of Possible Health Risk." Last modified January 3, 2011. http://www .fda.gov/Safety/Recalls/ucm238636.htm. Flynn, "Jimmy John's Permanently Dropping Sprouts from Menus."

5. CDC, "Multistate Outbreak of Human *Salmonella* I 4,[5],1 2:i: Infections Linked to Alfalfa Sprouts (FINAL Update)." Last modified February 10, 2011. Accessed January 2013. http://www.cdc.gov/salmonella/i4512i-/021011/.

6. CDC, "Investigation of an Outbreak of *Salmonella* Saintpaul Infections Linked to Raw Alfalfa Sprouts." Last modified May 2009. Accessed April 10, 2013.

7. "Boulder Sandwich Shop Closed over *E. coli* Outbreak." *Denver Channel*, October 9, 2008. Accessed January 2013. http://www.thedenverchannel.com/news/boulder-sandwich-shop-closed-over-e-coli-outbreak.

8. "The Ten Riskiest Foods Regulated by the U.S. Food and Drug Administration." Center for Science in the Public Interest. Accessed January 2013. http://cspinet.org/new/pdf/cspi_top_10_fda.pdf.

9. FoodSafety.gov, "Sprouts: What You Should Know." Accessed July 26, 2013. http://www.foodsafety.gov/keep/types/fruits/sprouts.html.

10. John Painter, CDC, "Attribution of Foodborne Illnesses, Hospitalizations, and Deaths to Food Commodities." http://wwwnc.cdc.gov/eid/article/19/3/11-1866_article.htm.

11. Glenn Morris, director, Emerging Pathogens Institute at the University of Florida, interview by Jennifer Brown, February 2013.

12. CDC, "Investigation Update: Multistate Outbreak of Human *Salmonella* Heidelberg Infections Linked to Ground Turkey." Last modified November 10, 2011. Accessed February 2013. http://www.cdc.gov/salmonella/heidelberg/111011/.

13. Cargill Meat Solutions, "Press Release on Recall." Last modified August 2011. Accessed February 2013. http://www.cargill.com/news/releases/2011/NA3047807.jsp.

14. CDC, "Multistate Outbreak of *Salmonella* Hadar Infections Associated with Turkey Burgers." Last modified April 2011. Accessed July 26, 2013. http://www.cdc.gov/salmonella/hadar0411/040411/.

15. Federal Register, "HACCP Plan Reassessment for Not-Ready-to-Eat Comminuted Poultry Products and Related Agency Verification Procedures." Last modified December 2012. Accessed April 9, 2013.

16. Jennifer Brown, "Concerns Grow over *Salmonella* That Survives Antibiotics." *Denver Post*, December 26, 2011.

17. Brown, "Concerns Grow over *Salmonella* That Survives Antibiotics."

18. Michael Batz, Sandra Hoffmann, and J. Glenn Morris Jr., Emerging Pathogens Institute, University of Florida. "Ranking the Risks: The 10 Pathogen-Food Combinations with the Greatest Burden on Public Health. 2011." Accessed April 10, 2013. http://www.epi.ufl.edu/sites/www.epi.ufl.edu/files/RankingTheRisks REPORT.pdf.

19. Batz et al., "Ranking the Risks."

20. Food Safety and Inspection Service, "FSIS Comparative Risk Assessment for *Listeria monocytogenes* in Ready-to-Eat Meat and Poultry Deli Meats." May 2010.

21. M.-S. Rhee, S.-Y. Lee, R. H. Dougherty, and D.-H. Kang, "Antimicrobial Effects of Mustard Flour and Acetic Acid against *Escherichia coli* O157:H7, *Listeria monocytogenes*, and *Salmonella enterica* serovar Typhimurium." *Applied and Environmental Microbiology* 69, no. 5 (2003).

22. Jennifer Brown, "Children's Illness Stirs Debate on Raw Milk." *Denver Post*, September 6, 2010.

23. Painter, "Attribution of Foodborne Illnesses, Hospitalizations, and Deaths to Food Commodities."

24. Dr. Patricia Griffin, chief of enteric diseases at the CDC's epidemiology office.

25. CDC, "Update on Multi-State Outbreak of *E. coli* O157:H7 Infections from Fresh Spinach, October 6, 2006." Last modified October 2006.

26. Indiana State Department of Health, "Taco John *E. coli* Outbreak." Last modified 2007. http://www.in.gov/isdh/24191.htm.

27. FDA, "Leafy Greens Safety Initiative Continues (2nd Year)." Last modified 2004. Accessed July 26, 2013. http://www.fda.gov/Food/FoodborneIllness Contaminants/BuyStoreServeSafeFood/ucm115898.htm.

28. FDA, "FDA: New Final Rule to Ensure Egg Safety, Reduce *Salmonella* Illnesses Goes into Effect." Last modified July 9, 2010.

29. Gardiner Harris. "Administration Issues New Rules on Egg Safety." *New York Times*, July 8, 2009. http://www.nytimes.com/2009/07/08/health/policy/08eggs .html?_r=2&scp=1&sq=egg rule&st=cse&.

30. "The Ten Riskiest Foods Regulated by the FDA."

31. Batz et al., "Ranking the Risks: The Ten Pathogen-Food Combinations with the Greatest Burden on Public Health."

32. CDC, "Toxoplasmosis." Accessed February 2013. http://www.cdc.gov/ parasites/toxoplasmosis/gen_info.

33. Painter, "Attribution of Foodborne Illnesses, Hospitalizations, and Deaths to Food Commodities."

34. "The Ten Riskiest Foods Regulated by the FDA."

35. CDC, "Multistate Outbreak of *Salmonella* Bareilly and *Salmonella* Nchanga Infections Associated with a Raw Scraped Ground Tuna Product." Last modified July 26, 2012. http://www.cdc.gov/salmonella/bareilly-04-12/.

36. Louisiana Department of Health, "DHH Recalls Oysters and Closes Oyster Harvesting Area." Last modified May 8, 2012. http://www.dhh.louisiana.gov/index .cfm/newsroom/detail/2484.

37. Center for Science in the Public Interest, "Gulf Coast Oyster Unsafe (But Not for the Reason You Think): Deadly *Vibrio vulnificus* Bacteria, Not Oil, Contaminate Gulf Oysters Every Summer." Last modified June 24, 2010. Accessed June 2010. http://cspinet.org/new/201006241.html.

38. Scott Harper, "FDA Warning Spurs Push for Stricter Oyster Rules." *Virginian-Pilot*, March 29, 2010. http://hamptonroads.com/2010/03/fda-warning -spurs-push-stricter-oyster-rules-va.

39. Painter, "Attribution of Foodborne Illnesses, Hospitalizations, and Deaths to Food Commodities."

40. Elaine Porterfield and Adam Berliant, "Jack in the Box Ignored Safety Rules." *News Tribune*, June 16, 1995. Accessed April 10, 2013. http://www.about-ecoli.com/ ecoli_outbreaks/news/jack-in-the-box-ignored-safety-rules/. Also, internal Jack in the

Box documents online. Last modified January 2013. Accessed July 26, 2013. http://www.foodsafetynews.com/2013/01/publishers-platform-lessons-learned -the-hard-way/.

41. "The Ten Riskiest Foods Regulated by the FDA."

42. Democratic Policy Committee, "Recent Food Safety Incidents in FDA Regulated Products." Accessed April 11, 2013. http://dpc.senate.gov/dpcdoc-safety timeline.cfm?doc_name=fs-111-2-58.

43. FDA, "Cal Fresco, LLC Recalls Jalapeño and Serrano Chili Peppers Due to Possible Health Risk." Last modified December 21, 2011. http://www.fda.gov/ Safety/Recalls/ucm284531.htm.

44. "S & P Company, Limited Recalls Su-nun Crush Roasted Thai Red Pepper Because of Possible Health Risk." Last modified October 12, 2012. http://www.fda .gov/Safety/Recalls/ucm323812.htm.

45. CDC, "Multistate Outbreak of *Salmonella* Typhimurium and *Salmonella* Newport Infections Linked to Cantaloupe." Last modified October 5, 2012. http:// www.cdc.gov/salmonella/typhimurium-cantaloupe-08-12/.

46. Michael Booth and Jennifer Brown, "Federal Agencies Try to Push Safe-Practice Guidelines, but Melons Still High-Risk." *Denver Post*, October 2, 2011. http://www.denverpost.com/recommended/ci_19022225.

47. G. Lopez-Velasco et al., "Assessment of Root Uptake and Systemic Vine-Transport of *Salmonella* enterica sv. Typhimurium by Melon (Cucumis melo) during Field Production." *International Journal of Food Microbiology* 158, no. 1 (2012). http://www.ncbi.nlm.nih.gov/pubmed/22824339.

CHAPTER 8

1. Thomas G. Neltner et al., "Navigating the U.S. Food Additive Regulatory Program." *Comprehensive Reviews in Food Science and Food Safety* 10, no. 6 (2011): 342–70.

2. Mark Lynas, "Lecture to Oxford Farming Conference." Last modified 2013. Accessed April 1, 2013. http://www.marklynas.org/2013/01/lecture-to-oxford -farming-conference-3-january-2013/.

3. Food and Water Watch, "Unseen Hazards: From Nanotechnology to Nano-toxicity." Last modified November 2009. Accessed February 2013. http://www .foodandwaterwatch.org/europe/questionable-technologies/nanotechnology/ unseen-hazards-view-in-full/.

4. Andrew Pollack, "Dow Corn, Resistant to a Weed Killer, Runs into Opposi-tion." *New York Times*, April 25, 2012.

5. Michael Specter, "The Seed Wars." *The New Yorker*, November 2, 2012.

6. G. Bruening and J. M. Lyons, "The Case of the Flavr Savr Tomato." *Califor-nia Agriculture* 54, no. 4 (2000): 6–7.

7. Ibid.

8. Kent Bradford, director, Seed Biotechnology Center, University of California, Davis, interviewed by Michael Booth, January 2013.

9. Monsanto, "Monsanto Company History." Accessed March 2013.

10. U.S. Government General Accounting Office, "Genetically Modified Foods: Experts View Regimen of Safety Tests as Adequate, but FDA's Evaluation Process Could Be Enhanced." Washington, D.C.: GAO, 2002.

11. American Association for the Advancement of Science, "Statement by the AAAS Board of Directors on Labeling of Genetically Modified Foods." Last modified October 2012.

12. Food Safety Department, World Health Organization, "Twenty Questions on Genetically Modified Foods." Accessed January 2013. http://www.who.int/food safety/publications/biotech.

13. Food Safety Department, World Health Organization, "Modern Food Biotechnology, Human Health and Development: An Evidence-Based Study." 2005. Accessed January 2013. http://www.who.int/foodsafety/publications/biotech/ biotech_en.pdf.

14. AAAS, "Statement."

15. Ibid.

16. Patty Lovera, assistant director, Food and Water Watch, interview by Michael Booth, January 2013.

17. Andrew Pollack, "Crop Scientists Say Biotechnology Seed Companies Are Thwarting Research." *New York Times*, February 19, 2009. Accessed August 2013.

18. Richard Brenneman, "Professor Ignacio Chapela Wins Bitter UC Tenure Fight." *The Berkeley Daily Planet*, May 24, 2005. Accessed August 2013.

19. Doug Gurian-Sherman, senior scientist, Food and Environment Program, interview by Michael Booth, February 2013.

20. Mark Bittman, "Buying the Vote on G.M.O.'s." *New York Times*, Opinionator, October 23, 2012.

21. Pollack, "Crop Scientists Say Biotechnology Seed Companies Are Thwarting Research."

22. Terry Etherton, head of the Department of Animal Science, Penn State University, interview by Michael Booth, January 2013.

23. Lynas, "Lecture to Oxford Farming Conference."

24. Patricia Hunt et al. (Letter from twenty-one concerned scientists), "Food Labels Would Let Consumers Make Informed Choices." Last modified 2012. http://www.environmentalhealthnews.org/ehs/news/2012/yes-labels-on-gm-foods.

25. European Commission, "Rules on GMOs in the EU." Accessed March 2013. http://ec.europa.eu/food/food/biotechnology/gmo_labelling_en.htm.

26. AAAS, "Statement."

27. Hunt et al., letter.

28. California Right to Know, "Media Briefing: Narrow Loss; Movement Victory—What's Next for GMO Labeling?" Last modified November 2012. Accessed April 2013. http://www.reuters.com/article/2012/11/07/idUS214455+07 -Nov-2012+PRN20121107.

29. Stephanie Strom, "Genetic Changes to Food May Get Uniform Labeling." *New York Times*, January 31, 2013.

30. Jerry Hagstrom, "Senators Offer Amendments to Ag Appropriations Bill." *AgWeek*, September 12, 2011. http://www.agweek.com/event/article/id/19068.

31. Center for Food Safety, "Genetically Engineered Fish, Food Safety Fact Sheet," January 2013. Accessed August 2013.

32. Josh Schonwald, *The Taste of Tomorrow* (New York: HarperCollins, 2012), 207.

33. William Muir et al., "Possible Ecological Risks of Transgenic Organism Release When Transgenes Affect Mating Success: Sexual Selection and the Trojan Gene Hypothesis." *Proceedings of the National Academy of Sciences* 96, 13853–56, November 23, 1999.

34. Brady Dennis, "Genetically Altered Salmon Are Safe, FDA Says." *Washington Post*, December 21, 2012.

35. Conservation Council, Alaska Marine et al. "Opposition to Approval of AquaBounty Genetically Modified Salmon." Last modified September 2010. Accessed April 2013. http://www.akmarine.org/ge-salmon-fishing-sign-on-letter.

36. Etherton, interview.

37. U.S. Food and Drug Administration, "Animal Cloning Risk Assessment." Last modified October 2009. Accessed April 1, 2013. http://www.fda.gov/Animal Veterinary/SafetyHealth/AnimalCloning/ucm055516.htm.

38. Etherton, interview.

39. U.S. FDA, "Animal Cloning Risk Assessment."

40. Michael T. Osterholm, "Foodborne Disease: The More Things Change, The More They Stay the Same." *Clinical Infectious Diseases* 39, no. 1 (2004): 8–10.

41. Robert V. Tauxe, "Food Safety and Irradiation: Protecting the Public from Foodborne Infections." *Emerging Infectious Diseases* 7, no. 3 Supplement (2001): 519.

42. Osterholm, "Foodborne Disease: The More Things Change."

43. Bill Marler, Marler Clark, "Pros and Cons of Commercial Irradiation of Fresh Iceberg Lettuce and Fresh Spinach: A Literature Review." Last modified December 2008. Accessed April 1, 2013. http://www.marlerblog.com/uploads/file/ProsandConsIRR.pdf.

44. Lisa Shames, U.S. General Accounting Office, "Federal Oversight of Food Irradiation." February 2010. Accessed April 1, 2013.

45. Lovera, interview.

46. Bill Marler, food safety attorney, Marler Clark, Seattle. Interview by Michael Booth, December 2011.

47. Beth Weiss, corporate communications director, Omaha Steaks. Interviewed by Michael Booth, February 2013.

48. Schonwald, *Taste of Tomorrow*, 263.

49. Jennifer Kuzma and Peter VerHage, *Nanotechnology in Agriculture and Food Production: Anticipated Applications*. Woodrow Wilson International Center for Scholars, Project on Emerging Nanotechnologies, September 2006.

50. Ibid., 9.

51. Food and Water Watch, "Unseen Hazards."

CHAPTER 9

1. Information on each pathogen in this chapter is gleaned from a variety of books, medical journals, expert interviews by the authors, diagnostic materials for medical professionals, federal agency food safety materials, and other works. A selected bibliography for this chapter includes: American Medical Association and Centers for Disease Control and Prevention et al., "*Escherichia coli* O157:H7 Infection, Patient Scenario," *Diagnosis and Management of Foodborne Illnesses* (2004); U.S. Food and Drug Administration, *Employee Health and Personal Hygiene Handbook* (Washington, D.C.: U.S. Government, 2005); American Medical Association and Centers for Disease Control and Prevention et al., "*Listeria monocytogenes* Infection, Patient Scenario," *Diagnosis and Management of Foodborne Illnesses: A Primer for Physicians* (2001); Division of Foodborne, Waterborne, and Environmental Diseases. Centers for Disease Control and Prevention, "Shigellosis: General Information." Last modified 2009. Accessed December 2012. http://www.cdc.gov/nczved/divisions/dfbmd/diseases/shigellosis; FoodSafety.gov. FDA, USDA/FSIS, CDC, "Food Poisoning: *Shigella*." Accessed December 2012; American Medical Association and American Nurses Association et al., "Acute Hepatitis A, Patient Scenario," *Diagnosis and Management of Foodborne Illnesses: A Primer for Physicians and Other Health Care Professionals* (2004); Benjamin Silk, Centers for Disease Control and Prevention, "*Listeria*: Food Poisoning's Rare but Deadly Germ." Last modified 2012. Accessed December 2012. www.cdc.gov/listeria/definition.html; Dr. Charles Patrick Davis, MD, MedicineNet.com, "*Salmonella* Poisoning." Last modified 2012. Accessed December 2012. www.medicinenet.com/script/main/art.asp?articlekey=85146; DynaMed. EBSCO Publishing, "*Salmonella ileocolitis*." Last modified November 26, 2012. Accessed January 2013. www.dynamed.ebscohost.com; DynaMed. EBSCO Publishing, "Norovirus Infection." Last modified December 5, 2012. Accessed January 2013. www.dynamed.ebscohost.com; Division of Foodborne, Waterborne, and Environmental Diseases. Centers for Disease Control and Prevention, "*Salmonella*." Last modified April 2012. Accessed January 2013. www.cdc.gov/salmonella/general/index.html; National Center for Immunization and Respiratory Diseases, Division of Viral Diseases. Centers for Disease Control and Prevention, "Norovirus." Last modified May 2012. Accessed January 2013. www.cdc.gov/norovirus/index.html; Aron J. Hall, "Noroviruses: The Perfect Human Pathogens?," *Journal of Infectious Diseases* (2012). Accessed December 2012. 10.1093/infdis/jis251; Aron J. Hall, DVM, Division of Viral Diseases, National Center for Immunization and Respiratory Diseases, Centers for Disease Control and Prevention, interview by Michael Booth, December 2012; Division of Foodborne, Waterborne, and Environmental Diseases. Centers

for Disease Control and Prevention, *"E. coli."* Last modified August 2012. Accessed January 2013. www.cdc.gov/ecoli/general/index.html; Division of Foodborne, Waterborne, and Environmental Diseases. Centers for Disease Control and Prevention, "Staphylococcal Food Poisoning." Last modified June 2010. Accessed December 2012. www.cdc.gov/nczved/divisions/dfbmd/diseases/staphylococcal; Division of Foodborne, Waterborne, and Environmental Diseases. Centers for Disease Control and Prevention, *"Campylobacter."* Last modified July 2010. Accessed December 2012. www.cdc.gov/nczved/divisions/dfbmd/diseases/campylobacter; DynaMed. EBSCO Publishing, "Enterohemorrhagic *Escherichia coli* infection." Last modified March 2012. Accessed January 2013. www.dynamed.ebscohost.com; DynaMed. EBSCO Publishing, *"Campylobacter enterocolitis."* Last modified July 2011. Accessed January 2013. www.dynamed.ebscohost.com; Michelle Barron, MD, division of Infectious Diseases, University of Colorado Hospital, interview by Michael Booth, March 2013; Louis M. Bell, MD, Mary Lou Manning, RN, Jane Brooks, and Marion Steinman, *The Children's Hospital of Philadelphia Guide to Common Childhood Infections* (New York: Macmillan, 1998); Carol A. Turkington, *Protect Yourself from Contaminated Food and Drink* (New York: Ballantine Books, 1999); Nicols Fox, *It Was Probably Something You Ate* (New York: Penguin Group, 1999); Morton Satin, *Food Alert! The Ultimate Sourcebook for Food Safety* (New York: Facts on File, 2008); Division of Foodborne, Waterborne, and Environmental Diseases. Centers for Disease Control and Prevention, "Giardiasis Frequently Asked Questions." Last modified July 2012. Accessed January 2013. www.cdc.gov/parasites/giardia/gen_info/faqs.html; Food and Drug Administration, "Bad Bug Book: Foodborne Pathogenic Microorganisms and Natural Toxins Handbook, *Clostridium perfringens."* Last modified 2012. Accessed January 2013. www.fda.gov/food/foodsafety/foodborneillness/Contaminants/CausesOfIllnessBadBugBook/ucm070483.htm; Division of Parasitic Diseases and Malaria. Centers for Disease Control and Prevention, "Toxoplasmosis Frequently Asked Questions." Last modified June 2011. Accessed January 2013. www.cdc.gov/parasites/toxoplasmosis/gen_info/faqs.html; Division of Foodborne, Waterborne, and Environmental Diseases. Centers for Disease Control and Prevention, *"Clostridium perfringens."* Last modified July 2011. Accessed January 2013. www.cdc.gov/foodborneburden/clostridium-perfringens.html; Division of Foodborne, Waterborne, and Environmental Diseases. Centers for Disease Control and Prevention, "CDC 2011 Estimates: Findings." Last modified October 2012. Accessed February 2013. www.cdc.gov/foodborneburden/2011-foodborne-estimates.html.

CHAPTER 10

1. Michael Doyle, director of the Center for Food Safety at the University of Georgia, interview by Jennifer Brown, March 2013.

2. David Lineback, senior fellow at the Joint Institute for Food Safety and Applied Nutrition at the University of Maryland, interview by Jennifer Brown, March 2013.

3. Jeff Nelken, food safety coach, interview by Jennifer Brown, March 2013.

4. U.S. Department of Health and Human Services, "Prevention of *Salmonella* Enteritidis in Shell Eggs during Production, Storage, and Transportation." *Federal Register* 74 (Thursday, July 9, 2009). Accessed April 17, 2013. http://www.gpo.gov/fdsys/pkg/FR-2009-07-09/pdf/E9-16119.pdf.

5. William Neuman, "U.S. Rejected Hen Vaccine Despite British Success." *New York Times*, August 24, 2010.

6. Ibid.

7. Michele Jay-Russell, program manager and research microbiologist at the Western Center for Food Safety at the University of California, interview by Jennifer Brown, March 2013.

8. Michele Jay-Russell and Michael Payne, "Are Free-Range Eggs Safer?" *CNN*, August 26, 2010. http://www.cnn.com/2010/OPINION/08/26/jay.russell.payne.eggs/index.html.

9. Dan Hale, professor of meat science at Texas A&M University, interview by Jennifer Brown, March 2013.

10. Cargill Press Release. Last modified August 3, 2011. http://www.cargill.com/news/releases/2011/NA3047807.jsp.

11. Mike Martin, Cargill Meat Solutions, interview by Jennifer Brown, March 2013.

12. CDC, "Final Report on Outbreak Investigation." Accessed April 17, 2013. http://www.cdc.gov/salmonella/heidelberg/111011/.

13. CDC, "Final Report."

14. Mike Martin, interview.

15. H. Russell Cross, head of the animal science department at Texas A&M University, interview by Jennifer Brown, March 2013.

16. International Food Safety Network, "Meat Thermometers, Not Color, Best Indicator for Doneness." Last modified December 21, 2000. Accessed April 17, 2013. http://foodsafety.k-state.edu/en/news-details.php?a=1&c=27&sc=221&id=20351.

17. "Public Health Alert." Last modified August 8, 2011. Accessed April 17, 2013. http://www.co.washington.or.us/HHS/News/strawberries.cfm.

18. Gretchen Goetz, "Did Deer Cause Oregon's Strawberry Outbreak?" *Food Safety News*, August 9, 2011.

19. Cookson Beecher, "Fresh Produce at Farmers Markets Exempt from New Food Safety Regs." *Food Safety News*, January 30, 2013.

20. Stanford University, "Little Evidence of Health Benefits from Organic Foods, Stanford Study Finds." Last modified September 3, 2012. http://med.stanford.edu/ism/2012/september/organic.html.

21. Kenneth Chang, "Stanford Scientists Cast Doubt on Advantages of Organic Meat and Produce." *New York Times*, September 3, 2012.

22. Chiemi Hayashi, "How Hubris Put Our Health at Risk." *CNN*, January 17, 2013. http://edition.cnn.com/2013/01/08/business/opinion-davos-hayashi-health.

23. National Resources Defense Council, "Raising Resistance: Feeding Antibiotics to Healthy Food Animals Breeds Bacteria Dangerous to Human Health." Last modified October 11, 2011. Accessed April 17, 2013. http://www.nrdc.org/health/raisingresistance.asp.

24. National Resources Defense Council, "Superbug Suit: Court Slams FDA on Antibiotics in Animal Feed . . . Again." Last modified June 5, 2012. http://www.nrdc.org/media/2012/120605.asp.

25. National Resources Defense Council, "Court Orders FDA to Address Antibiotic Overuse in Livestock and Protect Effectiveness of Medicine for Humans." Last modified March 23, 2012. http://www.nrdc.org/media/2012/120323.asp.

26. Liz Szabo and Peter Eisler, "CDC Sounds Alarm on Deadly, Untreatable Superbugs." *USA Today*, March 6, 2013. http://www.usatoday.com/story/news/nation/2013/03/05/superbugs-infections-hospitals/1965133/.

27. Michael Booth. "CDC Superbug Report Was No Surprise to University, Other Colorado Hospitals." *Denver Post*, March 7, 2013. Accessed April 17, 2013. http://blogs.denverpost.com/health/2013/03/07/cdc-superbug-report-was-no-surprise-to-university-other-colorado-hospitals/2811/.

28. Eat Wild, "Eating Grass-Fed Beef May Lower Your Risk of *E. coli* Infection." Accessed April 17, 2013. http://www.eatwild.com/foodsafety.html.

29. Sarah Klein, attorney at the Center for Science in the Public Interest, interview by Jennifer Brown, January 2013.

30. Michael Joseph, Mile High Organics founder and chief executive, interview by Jennifer Brown, March 2013.

INDEX

ABOUT THE AUTHORS

Michael Booth was the lead health care writer for *The Denver Post* and covered health, medicine, health policy, and politics throughout his twenty-five-year journalism career. He was part of the team that won the 2000 and 2013 Pulitzer Prizes for Breaking News. He has made frequent appearances on commercial and public television and radio, and has won the National Education Writers' Award, Best of the West, American Health Care Journalists honors, and other awards. He also co-led the coverage of the most deadly foodborne illness outbreak of the past century, the cantaloupe *Listeria* illnesses of 2011, with Jennifer Brown. Their coverage of the *Listeria* outbreak became the outline for a congressional committee's scathing report about what went wrong at the source farm and in the supply chain that sold the tainted melons.

Jennifer Brown is an investigative reporter with *The Denver* Post and has covered health, medicine, and health policy for the past decade. She was part of the team that won the 2013 Pulitzer Prize for Breaking News. Brown led the team covering the two-year debate over national health care reform in 2009 and 2010. She has worked at The Associated Press, *The Tyler Morning Telegraph* in Texas, and *The Hungry Horse News* in Montana, and has won a National Headliner Award, three Katie awards, and the 2013 Best of the West award for investigative journalism. Brown also has covered the Colorado legislature, the 2008 Democratic National Convention, and child welfare reform. She co-led the coverage of the most deadly foodborne illness outbreak of the past century, the cantaloupe *Listeria* illnesses of 2011, with Michael Booth.